Overcoming Candida

NUTRITIONAL AND MEDICAL APPROACHES

A Help Yourself Guide By Dr Sarah Brewer

Medilance Publishing

Overcoming Candida

About the Author Dr Sarah Brewer MSc (Nutr Med), MA (Cantab), MB, BChir, RNutr, MBANT, CNHC, FRSM qualified from Cambridge University with degrees in Natural Sciences, Medicine and Surgery. After working in general practice and hospital medicine, she gained a Master's degree in Nutritional Medicine from the University of Surrey. Sarah is one of the few licensed doctors who is also a Registered Nutritionist and a Registered Nutritional Therapist. She is the award winning author of over 60 popular self-help books, a columnist for Prima and Editor-in-Chief of Yourwellness magazine www.yourwellness.com. Follow her occasional nutritional Tweets at www.twitter.com/DrSarahB.

Medilance (Guernsey) Ltd
www.medilance.com

Contents

Chapter 1 Candida Essentials

Chapter 2 Nutritional Approaches

The 5Rs Approach
  Remove: Parasites, Food Intolerances
  Reintroduce: Sufficient Chewing, Fibre, Vitamins, Minerals,
          Acidity, Digestive Enzymes, Bile
  Re-Inoculate: 'Friendly' Probiotic Bacteria
  Repair: Vitamin D, Omega-3s, L-Glutamine, Aloe Vera, Cumin
  Rebalance
          Benefits Of An Alkaline Diet
          The Traditional Anti-Candida
          Avoiding Stress

Chapter 3 Nutritional Supplements

Vitamin C
Vitamin D
Biotin
Iron
Magnesium
Selenium
Zinc
Artichoke
Caprylic Acid
Co-Enzyme Q10
Cranberry
Curcumin
Echinacea
Garlic

CHAPTER 1

Candida Essentials

At the beginning of the twentieth century, Candida infection was rare. Now, it is a significant problem for many people who are plagued with recurrent attacks. Many researchers believe this is due to the widespread use of broad-spectrum antibiotics which, as well as eradicating unwanted bacterial infections, also disrupt the normal balance of healthy microbes in the body. Other factors include changing modern lifestyles (hormonal contraception, raised stress levels, low-temperature washing machine cycles, processed foods) and changes within the Candida yeasts themselves, making them more virulent.

There is also increasing recognition that Candida may trigger a hypersensitivity reaction that is thought to be linked to common health conditions such as irritable bowel syndrome and feeling tired all the time.

> ***Did you know?*** *Candida infection is also known as candidiasis, candidosis and moniliasis as well as 'thrush'.*

What Is Candida?

Candida is the name for a group of yeast-like fungi that live happily in or on the body of just about everyone. They exist in balance with other micro-organisms on the skin, in the intestines and sometimes in the mouth or genital tract - often without causing harm.

Altogether, around 200 different species of Candida exist, but only a third are capable of growing at human body temperature of 37 degrees Centigrade, and only a handful cause clinically significant symptoms. Of these, the most important is *Candida albicans* - named after the white plaques that form on mucus membranes in a well-established infection. The common name for Candida infection is thrush - presumably because the rash reminded early researchers of the breast of the speckled song bird.

> **Did you know?** *Candida albicans accounts for up to 75% of yeasts recovered from body sites of fungal infection.*

Candida yeasts belong to a large group of fungi that have mostly lost the art of sexual reproduction. They increase in numbers by putting out buds that break off to form new daughter cells.

When viewed under the microscope, Candida yeasts can appear in several different forms, as:
- large, round, thick-walled inactive resting spores
- active yeast cells that may be round, slipper or pear-shaped
- asexually reproducing yeast cells with budding daughter cells

- a collection of elongated buds and threads that remain attached to one another rather than breaking off
- cells with long, thread-like structures (germ tubes or hyphae)
- a network of interwoven threads (mycelium).

The simple cell forms are seen when Candida yeasts colonise the skin, mouth, gut or lower reproductive tract without causing symptoms. The thread forms (hyphae) can burrow between body cells, however, to literally invade the tissues and cause symptoms of Candida overgrowth.

What Are The Symptoms?

If Candida proliferates in large numbers, or starts to invade the tissues, it produces a variety of symptoms which can include:
- itching, often with a skin rash or visible white clumps
- soreness and redness
- painful, localised swelling or swollen regional glands
- brittle nails
- difficulty swallowing
- painful sex
- cystitis
- vaginal discharge
- lack of energy, weight loss plus many other symptoms.

Recurrent Candida now makes life a misery for countless numbers of people.

Where Is Candida Found?

Unlike other medically important fungi, *Candida albicans* is rarely found in environmental samples taken from the tops of volcanoes, wildernesses, frozen tundra or oceans. They are almost always found in close association with humans or other warm-blooded animals and passed on through close contact. However, they can survive in the atmosphere by entering a resting state similar to suspended animation. These spores can survive a variety of inhospitable conditions, including the low temperature (40 degrees C) laundry cycle of your washing machine.

Candida live in or on the body of just about every member of the population. In fact, like most people, you carry your own unique blend of Candida strains which will opportunistically cause problems when your natural immunity is lowered by illness (eg a cold), stress (eg exams) or through taking antibiotics.

Candida yeasts colonise almost all newborn babies within a month of birth. When normal, healthy adults with no obvious signs of infection are checked, Candida is detectable in:
- the mouth of up to 50%
- the oesophagus of 11%
- the skin creases of up to 80%
- rectal swabs of 30%
- the faeces of 80%
- vaginal swabs from 55% of women.

It's therefore not surprising that three out of four women experience vaginal thrush at least once in their life, and that some are plagued with never-ending recurrences.

In addition, Candida yeasts are found in the mouth of 76% of hospital patients, on the hands of 12% of doctors and nurses, and in up to 20% of infections affecting medical implants such as catheters and even heart valves.

What Triggers Candida Overgrowth?

Candida yeast cells change from the superficial 'harmless' cell form to the invading thread form when conditions are favourable. For optimum survival they like a warm, moist place with a relatively neutral to acid pH (4.5 - 7.5) and a temperature of 20 - 38 degrees C. In fact, these are the usual conditions normally found in the vagina and some parts of the gut. If your immune system is working normally, and you are not physically or emotionally stressed, your body usually keeps invasion at bay.

Even when conditions are not ideal, the yeast can still proliferate if:
• a particularly virulent strain of Candida is present
• local temperature, humidity or acid levels temporarily change to encourage Candida growth (eg after vigorous exercise, after using a vaginal douche or when taking antacid medications)

- circulating hormones (especially oestrogen) change (eg at certain times in the female menstrual cycle and during pregnancy)
- there is an imbalance of other micro-organisms that usually keep yeasts in check (eg after taking antibiotics)
- local carbohydrate levels (glycogen or glucose) increase, providing ideal growing conditions for fungal cells (eg diabetes, or changing secretions during the menstrual cycle)
- physical or mental stress lowers immunity (eg working long hours, surgery, trauma)
- immune cells become temporarily less efficient at fighting fungal infections (eg vitamin or mineral deficiencies or another illness such as a viral cold)
- natural immunity is suppress by medication (eg corticosteroids, chemotherapy, immune modulators)
- natural immunity is suppressed by a serious illness such as a cancer or AIDS.

Keeping Candida At Bay

Your immune system consists of millions of armed cells that patrol your body to prevent disease. To perform these functions, immune cells must correctly identify what is a normal part of you, and what is an undesirable invader.

Each of your cells carries unique identity tags on its surface that label it as part of you. Immune cells learn to recognise these tags during fetal development and generally leave them alone. Foreign cells such as Candida yeasts bear different cell markers - usually in the form of sugar-protein complexes (glycoproteins) that allow your immune cells to instantly mark them for destruction.

As well as displaying self-markers, your body cells continually break down worn-out, internal proteins and display some of these fragments on the cell surface. This communicates each cell's internal conditions to circulating immune cells. An infected cell therefore bears both a self-tag plus a foreign marker (eg a Candida protein) so the cell is recognised as undesirable and destroyed.

Cells involved in the immune response

Different types of immune cell work together to protect against Candida infection. These communicate with each other by secreting chemical messengers (cytokines) which attract other patrolling immune cells when an invader is detected.

Macrophages – whose name means 'big eater'- are long-lived scavenger cells that patrol the body for many months, engulfing unwanted tissue debris, dead or dying cells and foreign invaders. Once a macrophage identifies a bacterium, virus, yeast or infected body cell, it secretes cytokines that act like a chemical scream to attract other immune cells into the area. At the same time, the macrophage absorbs foreign proteins (antigens) from the unwanted cell onto its surface and presents these to circulating lymphocytes to super-stimulate them into action.

Neutrophils make up around 60% of circulating white blood cells and are commonly known as 'pus' cells. They only live for 6-20 hours but still play a vital role. When attracted into an area of infection by the cytokines secreted from other immune cells, they engulf smaller invading micro-organisms such as yeast cells, pulling them inside their cell membrane in a process known as phagocytosis. A lethal bag of chemicals (including toxic hydrogen peroxide) is then emptied onto the invader to kill it. With larger invaders such as candidal hyphae, neutrophils stick to their surface and release chemicals that damage the cells until they swell and burst. Neutrophils also carry receptors on their cell surface that interact with antibodies and special protein bombs called complement (described below) that punch holes in Candida cell walls.

Lymphocytes make up around 40% of circulating white blood cells. Three different types have different patterns of activity: *Natural Killer (NK) cells* are mainly concerned with killing abnormal body cells such as those infected with a virus or which have turned cancerous. Like a kamikaze pilot, an NK cell usually dies during its attack. *B-lymphocytes* produce antibodies aimed against a particular foreign protein (antigen). Some of these antibodies protrude from the surface of the B-lymphocyte rather like the weapons on a Dalek. Until it encounters its antigen, a B-lymphocyte patrols the body in an armed but inactive form known as a B-memory cell. When it encounters a foreign antigen it recognises, such as a Candida protein, it powers up and produces large numbers of its single, specific antibody. These active,

8

bristling lymphocytes are known as B plasma cells. Their activity is regulated by *T lymphocytes*, which control, encourage or inhibit their various activities. During activation, a B plasma cell divides repeatedly so you build up a sub-population of cells producing this one, particular type of antibody. Once the invasion is over, you have many more of this one, particular type of B-lymphocyte memory cell patrolling your body. If the same invader is re-encountered, your immune system responds more quickly and effectively, making it less easy for an organism to gain a second foothold. This mechanism usually helps to prevent recurrent Candida infections.

Antibodies – also called immunoglobulins - are present throughout your body fluids and are produced by activated B lymphocytes, each of which produces only one identical type of antibody. Each antibody consists of four protein chains linked together to form a Y-shaped molecule. When an antibody recognises a foreign antigen (eg a surface marker on a yeast cell) the open end of the Y-shaped antibody clamps onto the antigen to make the cellular equivalent of a citizen's arrest. The antibody tail sticks out behind and waits for help to arrive in the form of a macrophage, neutrophil, natural killer cell, cytotoxic T lymphocyte or a protein bomb (complement). This extra help homes in on the antibody-antigen complex and quickly destroys it. A type of antibody called IgA is secreted onto cell surfaces and is especially important in protecting against Candida infections.

Complement consists of around 20 different, circulating proteins that stick to an antigen-antibody complex in a specific sequence. As the different proteins link together and build up, they eventually form a powerful enzyme. This enzyme acts like a protein bomb that literally blows a hole in the side of a bacterium or yeast cell to kill it.

All these different lines of defence must be overcome before the Candida yeast cells that normally live happily in or on your body can invade your tissues to cause a symptomatic infection.

How You Suppress Candida

Most yeast infections are kept at bay by a fine balance between the activity of your immune system and the virulence (ability to cause disease) of the strains of Candida you possess. In most cases, Candida colonises your body in a benign form that remains harmless. It is only when your normal defences break down that Candida can switch to become a disease-causing organism. It is therefore classed as an 'opportunistic' infection.

Your skin

Your outer layer of skin forms a hardened (cornified) physical barrier against the outside world. It is made up of dead skin cells that are transformed into armoured plates of the tough protein, keratin. These plates are regularly sloughed and replaced, so that any yeast cells sticking to them are lost from the outer surface of your body. Fats (lipids) present in sweat and skin oils also inhibit Candida growth. A breach in the integrity of your skin, such as a scratch, burn, excessive moisture (maceration) or a skin disease such as eczema is usually needed before Candida can enter. This is why Candida infections are common in skin folds (eg nappy or sweat rash) as a combination of warmth, moisture and noxious secretions makes the skin boggy. For a similar reason, Candida infection may occur in people whose hands are often wet (eg dishwashers), in children who regularly suck their thumb, and in the warm humid conditions of your belly-button (with or without the protection of a tiny ball of fluff).

Your mucus membranes

The mucus membranes lining your mouth, gut, respiratory and genito-urinary tracts are less well defended than your outer skin and are therefore more susceptible to Candida infection. These body surfaces are warm, moist places - exactly the sort of sites where Candida loves to grow. Subtle changes in the local environment can tip the balance so that an invasive infection occurs.

In the mouth, some protection is provided by the continual flush of saliva which contains digestive enzymes (eg amylase), chemicals (eg histatins) and IgA antibodies that inhibit Candida growth.

Factors which increase the risk of oral yeast infections include having mouth ulcers, smoking cigarettes, wearing dentures, using inhaled corticosteroids to treat asthma or chronic obstructive pulmonary disease, and having a raised blood glucose level (diabetes).

> *Did you know?* *Sheer numbers of Candida cells can cause mouth infection. A volunteer who drank a solution containing a billion Candida cells developed Candidosis of the gut and live yeast cells were later isolated from his bloodstream and urine.*

Secretions in the oesophagus (gullet) and intestines also contain enzymes, antibodies and infection-fighting cells (macrophages, neutrophils, lymphocytes). Taking oral corticosteroid tablets, antibiotics or treatments to suppress stomach acid production can all increase the chance of Candida infection taking hold. Similarly, using inhaled steroids can promote oesophageal candidiasis.

> *Did you know?* *Rinsing your mouth after using a corticosteroid inhaler reduces the chance of developing oral and oesophageal Candida, as does having a good inhaler technique.*

Tissue fluids

Once your skin or mucus membrane barrier is breached by Candida cells, your next line of defence consists of the immune factors present in your tissue fluids (your internal sea). These include immune cells, antibodies and the complement proteins that link up to punch holes in yeast cells. However, the presence of too many IgA antibodies may coat yeast cells so well that they become hidden from attacking immune cells. Paradoxically, this may help to keep the infection going. Some people also develop an allergic response to yeast cells, making a type of antibody called IgE which can make the symptoms associated with candidiasis worse.

Immune cells

Your most important final line of defence against Candida infection consists of the pus cells (neutrophils) and other scavengers (macrophages in the tissues, monocytes in your blood) that roam around your body, hunting and attacking invaders. These release chemicals that damage yeast cells, interfere with their metabolism (eg by binding zinc) and attract other immune cells into the area. Lack of neutrophils (eg in leukaemia) or reduced neutrophil function (due to inherited enzyme defects) increases the risk of developing widespread candidiasis.

Inflammation

Many of the symptoms associated with an attack of oral or vaginal thrush are due to the inflammatory reactions triggered by your immune defences. When patrolling macrophages encounter fungal hyphae, they start attacking the invaders and send out chemical alarm signals (cytokines) to attract other macrophages, neutrophils and lymphocytes into the area. Circulating antibodies also bind to Candida hyphae and attract immune cells and complement proteins to ramp up the immune response.

Tissue damage caused by Candida enzymes, and the chemicals released by your immune cells to fight the infection, cause tiny underlying blood vessels (capillaries) to dilate. Clear fluid (plasma) seeps from your blood into the area bringing in extra complement protein and antibodies, while separation of cells in the capillary wall makes it easier for immune cells to slip through into infected tissue. It's this dilation of blood vessels – a necessary part of your immune response – that causes the increased warmth, redness and swelling which accompanies inflammation. These chemicals also irritate nerve endings to cause pain – nature's way of alerting you that something is wrong. This is why Candida infections are so uncomfortable.

Allergic reactions

Some people are particularly sensitive to Candida infections due to circulating IgE antibodies that respond to Candida proteins. IgE triggers the release of histamine and other allergy chemicals from cells. Some T-lymphocytes over-react to the presence of yeast cells in a delayed hypersensitivity response that increases inflammation to cause excessive redness, swelling and pain. These abnormal immune reactions have been associated with feelings of tiredness all the time and lack of energy (See Candida Hypersensitivity Syndrome).

How Candida Strikes

There is evidence that some Candida yeasts alter your normal immune responses that keep them at bay. Substances present in *Candida albicans* cell walls, and which are released by their hyphae, can damp down the activity of neutrophils (pus cells) so they become:

- more sluggish
- less easily attracted into the area
- less able to engulf and absorb fungal proteins or cells

- less able to secrete toxic chemicals
- less responsive to certain bacterial infections.

Other fungal products appear to impair the activity of T-lymphocytes so they react less strongly to the present of Candida cells, allowing long-term (chronic) infections to occur.

To cause the symptoms of a thrush 'attack', Candida yeasts must evade your normal immune defences and invade body tissues.

Sticking

Candida yeast cells can stick to the lining of your mouth, gut, vulva or vagina. They do this using special receptors on their outer cell wall (the so-called fuzzy coat) that act rather like NASA landing gear, equipped with suckers. Their ability to stick depends on local conditions – they especially like warm, moist, neutral to acid conditions.

Growing

Once yeast cells obtain a firm anchorage, they put out germ tubes (hyphae) when conditions are right. These hyphae grow over the surface of surrounding host cells. As Candida yeast cells bud, divide and increase their number, more hyphae are produced. Eventually the colony forms a raised, white plaque resembling a curd of cottage cheese.

Dissolving

Hyphae secrete enzymes that break down your cell proteins (eg collagen) and fats (eg lipid membranes). These enzymes loosen and dissolve the connections between cells, letting the hyphae burrow down to invade your tissues. The hyphae tips can even sneak inside your cells to steal the nutrients and energy they need to fuel their continuing growth. This enzyme activity is responsible for some of the soreness and inflammation that accompanies an attack of thrush. *Candida albicans* cells produce more of these enzymes than other Candida species, which is why they cause the most troublesome yeast infections.

Switching

In the laboratory, colonies of Candida yeast cells growing in culture plates have a smooth, rounded surface. When exposed to ultraviolet light, they switch to producing colonies with an uneven, rough surface. These switched (rough) colonies produce germ tube threads (hyphae) that:
- stick to body lining cells more easily
- proliferate more readily
- secrete more enzymes to break down proteins, fats and cell membranes
- are more invasive
- more easily escape immune detection
- are less susceptible to anti-fungal treatments.

This is especially likely to happen when Candia yeasts on your body are exposed to sunlight or UV sunbeds.

16

Secretion of virulence factors

Switching and increased invasiveness of Candida yeasts is usually associated with the production of one or more virulence factors. These allow yeasts to stick more firmly to your cells (adhesion factors) or secrete more aggressive enzymes (eg aspartate proteinases and phospholipases) to either penetrate your tissues more easily, or inactive your antibody or other defences. Gliotoxin, for example, is produced by some Candida strains to impair immune cell activity. Some Candida yeasts also produce factors that let them swarm over surfaces to form three-dimensional biofilms. These factors surround them like a protective cocoon, helping them escape immune attacks and antifungal drugs. Some yeast cells reduce their production of a membrane building block, called ergosterol, which reduces their sensitivity to some antifungal drugs (eg terbinafine) by thirty to two thousand fold. Other yeasts have acquired so-called membrane efflux pumps which expel antifungal drugs so they don't accumulate inside to kill them. A few Candida yeast strains have even evolved an ability to hide inside host cells, including immune scavenger cells (macrophages), where they survive unharmed.

17

Translocation

The gut is the main site from which Candida yeasts enter the body. Passing from the gut into the tissues is known as translocation (moving across). Live yeast cells can enter the circulation from anywhere in the bowel but this most usually happens in a part of the small intestines called the jejunum. When only a small number of yeast cells enter the circulation, they are normally mopped up by macrophage scavenger cells. When large numbers of Candida cells are involved, or where the immune system is weakened (for example by a cancer or HIV), the Candida yeasts may escape to spread throughout the body. Candida can also enter the circulation from the lungs, but this is thought to account for less than 3% of systemic Candida infections.

Invasion

When the immune system is suppressed, Candida can establish colonies deep in body tissues to form micro-abscesses. These can cause potentially lethal problems such as Candidal brain abscess, meningitis or fungus ball pneumonia which, thankfully, are all rare.

Predisposing factors

A number of factors can increase your risk of developing Candida symptoms. These include:
- Exposure to large numbers of Candida yeast cells
- Taking broad-spectrum or long-term antibiotics
- Experiencing excessive physical or emotional stress

- The presence of another infection that weakens your immune response (eg influenza, HIV)
- Reduced levels of acidity (pH 6 -8 for example, reduced stomach acid production, or vaginal changes following menstruation)
- Taking drugs to suppress stomach acid production (eg antacids)
- Short-term tissue damage (eg cuts, burns, mouth ulcers, tooth extraction)

Some other factors appear to increase the risk of experiencing recurrent Candida infections. These include:
- Having an immature or aged immune system (eg newborn infants, the elderly)
- Experiencing hormone fluctuations (eg pregnancy, menstrual cycle, menopause)
- Having a low ferritin level (indicating poor iron stores)
- Having a raised blood glucose level due to undiagnosed or poorly-controlled diabetes
- Lack of certain nutrients (protein, vitamins, minerals) needed for normal immunity
- Using inhaled corticosteroids (eg for asthma, chronic obstructive pulmonary disease)
- Long-term tissue damage (eg inflammatory bowel disease, bowel surgery, radiotherapy)
- Having an illness that weakens your general immunity (eg adrenal dysfunction, cancer, AIDS)
- Taking drugs that suppress immunity (eg oral corticosteroids, chemotherapy)

- Pronounced weight loss (eg elderly, extreme dieting, anorexia nervosa)
- Smoking cigarettes
- Excessive alcohol intake
- Wearing poorly fitting dentures, or poor oral hygiene
- Being bedridden
- Having an indwelling catheter, intravenous central line, heart valves or other prostheses.

Symptoms And Signs Of Candida

So many symptoms can be triggered by Candida - either through an overgrowth of the yeasts, or through hypersensitivity reactions to their presence - that it's easy for a sufferer to be dismissed by their doctor, family and colleagues as suffering from hypochondria or other neurosis. This is especially true if symptoms come and go or if they change, as they often do.

While some people only suffer mild, nuisance symptoms that do not interfere unduly with their life, others are debilitated by constant tiredness and non-specific feelings of being unwell. This interferes with concentration and can make you so irritable and depressed that it jeopardises relationships at home and at work.

What causes the symptoms of Candida overgrowth?

When Candida yeasts change from their simple cell form to the active invasive form, fungal threads (germ tubes or hyphae) burrow between the cells lining your mouth, gut, vagina, the end of the penis or around the anus. This causes small areas of ulceration and fissuring that exposes tiny, sensitive nerve endings. Some of the threads punch straight through your cells, releasing powerful intra-cellular enzymes into the surrounding tissues. This starts an inflammatory response which attracts immune cells into the area. These immune cells secrete more chemicals into your already inflamed tissues, blood vessels dilate and the area becomes increasingly red, hot, sore and swollen. These chemicals irritate raw nerve endings so you experience varying degrees of pain and throbbing depending on the severity of the infection. Local lymph nodes (glands) may also swell – for example in the groin if you have vaginal Candidosis.

As well as specific symptoms linked to the site of infection, you may also develop non-specific symptoms that are linked with Candida Hypersensitivity Syndrome (see later).

Could You Have Undiagnosed Diabetes?

Recurrent Candida can be a sign of raised blood glucose levels. One in ten adults, world-wide, lives with diabetes and numbers are increasing although at least half of cases remain undiagnosed.
Diabetes results from producing insufficient insulin hormone within the pancreas (type 1 diabetes) or an inability to respond to the insulin hormone produced (type 2 diabetes, associated with

obesity). The symptoms of type 1 and type 2 diabetes can include any or all of the following:

Symptoms of diabetes	Type 1	Type 2
Excessive thirst	YES	Unusual but can occur
Excessive drinking	YES	Unusual but can occur
Weight loss, despite hunger and increased eating	YES	Weight gain and obesity are more common
Tiredness, listlessness and fatigue	YES	Possible
Feeling unwell	Often	Unusual, but can occur
Recurrent Candida, cystitis or boils	YES	YES
Blurred vision	Often	Unusual but can occur

If you think you could have diabetes, contact your doctor as soon as possible.

Candida Skin Infections

A variety of yeasts and fungi cause skin infections, with symptoms varying from single scaly patches to widespread dry rashes or moist, boggy areas – especially in skin folds. Single lesions are often known as ringworm as they form a ring with a raised edge that spreads outwards as the centre clears. There is no worm involved however, only a fungus such as Pityrosporum yeasts and fungi known as Dermatophytes.

Candida skin infections typically cause redness and soreness rather than ringworm, and usually only occur if the skin is damaged by a build-up of moistness (eg in skin folds), burns, friction from tight, chaffing clothes or an existing skin problem such as eczema. Skin folds are most usually affected, such as:

• under the breasts
• in the groin, armpits or between the buttocks
• under rolls of fat on the abdomen
• in the belly button
• around the scrotum or penis
• around the vaginal entrance (vulvovaginitis)
• in the nappy area of babies.

Candida skin infections are especially common in infants, people with diabetes, those taking antibiotics, the overweight, and in the elderly. The symptoms of Candida skin infection may include any or all of the following:

• itching, soreness or redness
• a scaly, flaky or flat, red rash with scalloped edges
• acne-like spots or weeping sores
• a moist breakdown of skin (maceration)
• small satellite lesions spreading away from main area

• a build-up of white clots in skin folds.

Treatment

Candida skin infections usually respond quickly to antifungal creams, many of which are available over the counter from pharmacies (See Chapter 4). If there is significant inflammation, a combined anti-fungal and anti-inflammatory (corticosteroid) cream will reduce soreness more quickly. If the area is very moist (eg in an armpit or under the breasts), an anti-fungal powder can be used separately, or applied after the cream.

Other skin conditions can be mistaken for fungal infections. These include eczema, psoriasis, and even some forms of skin cancer (eg squamous cell carcinoma). If you think you have a fungal skin infection which has not responded to treatment within a couple of weeks, or which seems to be getting worse rather than better, it is important to seek medical advice.

> *Did you know?* *If a fungal skin infection is mistaken for eczema, and only a plain corticosteroid cream used to treat it (eg 1% hydrocortisone, betamethasone) a condition known as tinea incognita (hidden fungal infection) can occur. The steroid cream damps down redness, scaling and itching so the lesions feel better, but the underlying fungal infection continues to thrive. The skin lesion persists and grows larger - sometimes quite quickly. As soon as treatment is stopped, the infection will return with a vengeance. It is only when an anti-fungal agent is used that the skin infection improves. If in doubt about the diagnosis or treatment, always seek medical advice.*

24

Prevention

Aim to lose any excess weight to reduce skin folds.

Wash, shower or bathe every day to remove acidic, sweaty secretions from skin folds. Dry your skin thoroughly after wetting (if necessary, use a hairdryer on low heat to blow dry skin folds.

Wear loose clothes that allow air to circulate - avoid tight jeans, cycling shorts, jockey-style briefs and so on.

Select underpants/boxers made from cotton rather than man-made fibres.

Use an anti-fungal powder/spray in skin folds prone to excessive sweating.

Reduce excessive sweating eg use an aluminium hexahydrate anti-perspirant (but don't apply to infected skin or it will burn).

Don't share bath towels, flannels or bath sponges.

Candida And Male Infections

The groin is a warm, moist, sweaty area that harbours a variety of bacteria and yeasts. Candida infection of the male genitals is therefore common, especially in warm conditions such as summer months, holidays abroad or after exercise when sweat is allowed to remain in place afterwards.

Candida yeast infection is the most common problem to affect the tip of the penis and is known as balanitis. Inflammation around the foreskin is called posthitis, and when both occur together - which they frequently do - the result is known as balanoposthitis.

Balanitis affects up to 5% of young boys, usually striking before school age. Older males can also be affected – especially if a sexual partner carries Candida yeasts (with or without symptoms).

Mild Candidal balanitis causes mottled red spots, slight soreness and itching of the tip of the penis. There may also be a build-up of yeasty smegma under the foreskin. If the condition is left untreated and becomes worse, the skin may break down to leave weeping areas, a sticky discharge and painful swelling of the foreskin. This can lead to difficulty passing urine and enlargement of lymph nodes (glands) in the groin.

Always seek medical advice, as other causes of balanitis include infection with common skin bacteria, sexually transmissible diseases, allergic reactions to soap or bath additives and chemical irritation (eg nappy rash in babies). Swabs are usually sent for examination to confirm whether the infection is due to yeasts, bacteria or both. Urinalysis to check for glucose is important to rule out diabetes, in which balanitis is often one of the first signs in men.

Treatment

A study involving 43 men with mild balanitis showed that just washing the penis with water alone is often enough for symptoms to disappear without the need for further treatment. Don't use soap as this causes irritation and changes skin acidity, making the inflammation and infection worse.

Moderate to severe Candida balanitis will need medical assessment to exclude a bacterial infection or an underlying factor such as an over tight foreskin, or diabetes, which promotes yeast infection. If Candida is confirmed (by swabs for culture or examination under a microscope) treatment with a topical antifungal cream or gel is less greasy than an ointment and will feel more comfortable. If you are very sore, however, an ointment provides a barrier layer that protects skin from contact with urine and stale sweat. You may also find it helpful to use an anti-fungal powder spray around the groin, scrotum and tops of the legs to keep the area clean, dry and to prevent the infection spreading under cover of the warmth and humidity of your underpants.

If balanitis is severe with gross swelling of the foreskin, or if it is recurrent, circumcision may be necessary.

Prevention

Balanitis is preventable through good hygiene and frequent washing under the foreskin. In mild cases, simple bathing with salt water (saline) twice per day will quickly help symptoms resolve.

27

Did you know? Some cases of balanitis are also due to detergent allergy or irritation.

When bathing baby boys, the foreskin should never be forcibly retracted - in 96% of male babies, the foreskin is still attached to the front the glans penis and forcing it open can cause tissue damage, bleeding and scarring. The natural adhesions break down over the first few years of life - except for the normal attachment underneath, the frenulum - until by the age of three, 90% of foreskins are partially separated. Tissues remnants may remain up until adolescence however.

Boys over the age of 7 years who have not been circumcised, and whose foreskin can be gently retracted, should be taught how to wash underneath the foreskin at least once a day - and preferably after every urination. After washing, it is important to ensure the foreskin is pulled forward again to cover the tip of the penis. If it is left pulled back, its blood supply may become restricted leading to swelling (paraphimosis).

Although Candida is not necessarily sexually transmitted, it is a sexually transmissible disease, which means it can be passed on during sex, although this isn't the only or main way in which it is contracted.

Avoid intercourse until symptoms have disappeared as you can pass the infection on to your partner. Alternatively - assuming your symptoms aren't too unpleasant - use a condom together with the spermicide, nonoxynol-9, which has some anti-fungal action.

Candida And Female Infections

The vulva is the visible, external female genitalia and inflammation of the vulva is known as vulvitis. As the vagina is directly connect to the vulva, inflammation of the vulva usually spreads to involve the vagina too, so soreness in this area is usually referred to medically as vulvovaginitis.

The vagina is the most efficient self-cleansing organ in the body, and a certain amount of vaginal discharge is both natural and inevitable. A healthy discharge is relatively light rather than profuse, non-irritant, a white or buff colour and slightly acidic with a fresh smell that is not offensive.

Vaginal discharge contains infection fighting neutrophils (pus cells), antibodies and lactobacilli bacteria that secrete natural antifungal substances and weak acids (eg lactic acid) that help to discourage Candida overgrowth. Because of these suppressive factors, Candida is normally a harmless commensal organism that lives in the vagina without causing symptoms.

When vaginal swabs are grown in cultures, Candida yeasts are detected in between 10% to 55% of apparently well women with no symptoms of thrush infection. The average seems to be around 1 in 5 (20%). The yeast cells are either present in an inactive state (resting spores) or as simple cells (non-filamentous forms) in relatively small numbers, without hyphae. They are able to survive on the surface of vaginal lining cells but not to invade, and are shed regularly when the cell to which they are attached is shed.

Whether yeast cells come-and-go, or are present all the time, is not really known. Some studies suggest that Candida can remain in the vagina for at least several months, and possibly for years at a time without causing obvious harm. If the natural balance is tipped however - due to changing levels of hormones, acidity, sugar content or the numbers and types of bacteria present - Candida cells may suddenly proliferate to cause classic symptoms that can include:

- itching
- redness, soreness or burning
- vaginal dryness
- a white, cottage-cheese-like discharge
- yeast-like odour
- pain on intercourse
- cystitis-like pain on passing urine (dysuria)
- frequency of urination
- enlarged lymph nodes (glands) in the groin.

The amount of discharge does not necessarily relate to the severity of symptoms, and some women find that dryness makes their symptoms worse.

Other causes of itching and soreness that may be confused with Candida infection include bacterial imbalances (anaerobic vaginosis), Herpes simplex virus (cold sores), wart (papilloma) virus, allergy to chemicals in toiletries (deodorants, bath products, soaps, spermicides, creams, douches, lubricants), a lack of oestrogen around and after the menopause (atrophic vulvovaginitis), skin changes linked with ageing (vulval dystrophies), urinary irritation (eg stress incontinence) and skin problems such as eczema or psoriasis that can affect this area as well as other parts of the body. Simple itching alone may be caused by infestations such as pubic lice, scabies, or threadworms.

> **Important**: *Candida spores can survive under the male foreskin without causing problems. If you have recurrent Candida, ask your partner to use an anti-fungal cream and use condoms to see if this helps.*

Candida and vaginal acidity

The acidity of vaginal secretions changes throughout your menstrual cycle. For most of the month, secretions are acidic. This partly results from acids secreted by your own vaginal cells, but most are produced by friendly bacteria such as Lactobacillus acidophilus. As your period approaches, hormone changes make your vaginal discharge less acidic. Blood itself is slightly alkaline and during menstruation this makes the vaginal environment significantly less acidic. This also affects the friendly Lactobacilli present in vaginal secretions so that, under the microscope, they start to look larger, paler and more blotchy rather than the more normal thick, compact, dark-staining rods. They are struggling to survive due to the loss of acidity, and their reduced activity means

31

it is easier for Candida to proliferate rather than remaining in check.

When conditions are acidic, Candida tends to stay in its less invasive form as simple yeasts cells that occasionally bud and divide. When conditions are less acidic, they tend to produce the invasive threads (germ tubes, or hyphae) that trigger infection and symptoms. This switch from a simple celled form to the thread form occurs at around pH6 (just below neutral) and can happen within one to three hours of environmental conditions changing. As a result, vaginal candidiasis is more common just before, during and after your period.

> ***Did you know?*** *An acid gel (0.9% acetic acid in a jelly base) is available from pharmacies to help maintain vaginal acidity and encourage Candida cells to remain in their simple, non-invasive form.*

Glucose content of vaginal discharge and Candida

During the second half of your menstrual cycle (after ovulation) hormone changes increase the glycogen content of vaginal cells. Glycogen is a starchy storage compound that is broken down within cells to provide glucose sugar for energy – and as bakers and brewers know well, glucose is the favourite fuel for developing yeast cells. So, along with the tailing off of acidity that naturally occurs around the time of menstruation, there is also a slight increase in the level of glucose naturally present in vaginal cells and secretions, to increase the chance of developing thrush.

Women with undiagnosed or poorly treated diabetes also have increased glucose levels within their vaginal secretions, and many new cases of diabetes are identified following a severe attack of Candida vulvo-vaginitis.

Contraceptive hormones and vulvovaginal Candida

The synthetic hormones used in some forms of contraception can affect vaginal discharge and acidity, depending on the blend used.

Hormone treatments that are predominantly oestrogenic (contain relatively more oestrogen than progestogen) encourage increased vaginal secretions that are thin, elastic and sometimes copious. This is partly because they increase the number of mucus-secreting cells found around the cervix. Oestrogens also increase the stickiness of vaginal cells so that Candida yeasts find it easier to latch hold, and stimulate the production of yeast hyphae so that infection spreads more quickly.

Hormone treatments that are relatively progestogenic (contain relatively more progestogen than oestrogen) produce the opposite effect - scant, thick mucus that is accompanied by vaginal dryness.

Taking synthetic hormones is also known to affect the glycogen content of vaginal cells, to increase the risk of developing vulvo-vaginal Candida. This is most likely if the hormone blend you are on contains relatively high doses of oestrogen. Blends containing low doses of oestrogen are less likely to cause problems with vulval or vaginal thrush.

If you are using a hormonal method of contraception and experience recurrent thrush, talk to your doctor about whether changing your method of contraception may help.

Pregnancy and vulvovaginal Candida

Around one in three women develop symptoms of vulvovaginal thrush at least once during pregnancy. Thrush is most likely to strike during the last three months of pregnancy, and recurrences are common.

Pregnancy is a time when natural immunity is lowered so the developing baby's foreign genes, inherited from their father, are not attacked by the mother's defences. The pregnancy hormone, progesterone, damps down the growth and proliferation of white blood cells (lymphocytes) that produce antibodies, for example.

Significantly raised oestrogen levels increase the glycogen content of vaginal cells, and pregnancy is also a time when sugar-handling is increasingly impaired, so that sugar levels throughout the body are higher than normal. This provides more fuel for the growth and division of any Candida yeasts present.

High levels of oestrogen hormone increase the stickiness of vaginal cells so that Candida yeasts are more likely to bind to them, and stimulate the production of Candida hyphae so that a yeast infections spreads more quickly.

34

Antibiotics and vulvovaginal Candida

Many women notice that Candida symptoms develop during or after a course of antibiotics. The most common culprits are broad-spectrum antibiotics (eg tetracycline, ampicillin, amoxycillin, cephalosporins) that wipe out the healthy bacteria found in the vagina and gut as well as the disease causing bacteria they are designed to treat.

These healthy bacteria (especially Lactobacillus) keep Candida at bay be competing for nutrients, binding sites on vaginal lining cells and by secreting chemicals that increase local acidity and inhibit yeast growth. Studies show that Candida is three times more likely to be found in the vagina of women taking antibiotics than those not taking them, although they do not necessarily always cause symptoms.

Taking a probiotic supplement will help to replenish Lactobacilli in the gut, some of which find their way into the vagina. Some women like to smear the vulva with natural bio yoghurt containing live Lactobacillus acidophilus as these bacteria can colonise the vagina and help to prevent. While messy, this can be effective. Probiotic pessaries are also available.

Iron deficiency and vulvovaginal Candida

White blood cells need iron to make some of the powerful chemicals they use to combat infections. Even a mild iron deficiency, that is not sufficient to reduce production of the red blood pigment, haemoglobin, to cause iron-deficiency anaemia, can suppress immunity against Candida. So, even if your blood count (haemoglobin concentration) is normal, recurrent Candida could still be due to a low iron reserve. This is diagnosed by measuring blood levels of an iron-binding protein called ferritin.

> **Did you know?** *Ferritin is the main way in which iron is stored and transported around the body. It is made up of a protein, apoferritin, linked to a varying number of iron atoms - one molecule of apoferritin may contain as many as 4500 atoms of iron. When iron stores are low, less apoferritin is made and iron in the blood stream moves from apoferritin to another iron-transporting protein, transferrin.*

Ideally, all women with recurrent Candida should have their ferritin level measured. If low, treatment with an iron-containing vitamin and mineral supplement often solves the problem, although treatment needs to be continued for several months until iron stores return to normal. If you have a low ferritin level, you and your doctor will need to identify why your iron levels are low:

- Do you eat sufficient iron containing foods? (See Chapter 2)
- Do you have heavy or frequent periods?
- Have your iron stores been depleted through pregnancy?
- Are you losing hidden blood from your bowels?
- Is there a problem with iron absorption from your diet?
- Is there a problem with production of red blood cells in your bone marrow?

If the iron deficiency is significant, you will need investigations to determine the cause.

Tight clothes and vulvo-vaginal Candida

Wearing tight underclothes - especially those fashioned from man-made fibres that are unable to 'breathe' – greatly increases your risk of vulvovaginal Candida. Yeast spores are everywhere in the air, and love to germinate in warm, moist places so wearing tight clothes promotes ideal warm, humid conditions.

If you suffer from recurrent vulvovaginal thrush, wear loose, well-ventilated clothes and cotton underwear. Avoid nylon tights, and instead wear stockings - either those with elasticated tops that stay up on their own, or with a suspender belt for support.

Low-temperature wash cycles and Candida

In olden days, underwear received a thorough boil-up in a pan of water, on top of the stove, once a week. In contrast, modern wash-day practices involve environmentally-friendly low-temperature (eg 30 to 40 degrees C) wash cycles that protect delicate lingerie but do not kill Candida spores. They survive the process and may linger in your underwear to cause reinfection next time you wear that item of clothing. To prevent this, do one of the following: Continue washing your lingerie as before, but iron cotton gussets with a very hot iron to kill any residual Candida spores; pre-soak your underwear in concentrated detergent and scrub the crotch before putting them into the wash; wear white cotton underwear that can survive a hot wash (eg 90 degrees C) without undue damage, or soak your undies in bleach (it the material will take it) before washing. These measures are often enough to break the misery of a recurrent thrush re-infection cycle.

Sun beds and vulvo-vaginal Candida

Using a sun bed can trigger thrush, partly due to the increased warmth and moistness generated under the lamps, but also because ultra-violet light changes Candida yeasts from a relatively benign to a more virulent form.

As far back as the 1950s, it was noticed that when cells from a smooth colony of Candida yeasts were inoculated onto a new culture plate, a proportion developed into colonies with a rough, uneven surface that grew more quickly. This change was referred to as 'switching' but no-one was very excited by it. More recently, the phenomenon attracted new interest when it was discovered that switching could be triggered by exposing colonies to low doses of ultraviolet light.

Switched (rough) colonies produce different patterns of germ tube threads (hyphae) that:
- proliferate more readily
- stick to body lining cells more easily
- secrete more enzymes that break down proteins, fats and cell walls
- are more invasive
- escape detection by immune cells more easily
- are less susceptible to anti-fungal treatments.

Using a sun bed may therefore trigger symptoms of thrush in someone who has previously lived quite happily with their Candida without developing symptoms.

Avoid sun beds if you suffer from recurrent candidiasis (and even if you don't as they increase the risk of skin cancer). Artificial tanning techniques are widely available if you like a bronzed look.

Prevention summary

Avoid tight underwear, especially nylon pantyhose or tight trousers. Stockings and cotton underwear are best as they allow air to circulate, so that warmth and humidity are lower.

Avoid getting hot and sweaty - use panty-liners and change them as necessary throughout the day; shower, wash or bathe immediately after exercise.

Don't use bath additives, vaginal deodorants or douches - they can upset your natural acid and bacterial balance.

Avoid trauma to vaginal tissues from vigorous sex or rubbing too hard with a bath towel.

Try boiling cotton underwear or hot-ironing panty gussets. Modern low-temperature washing machine cycles don't kill Candida spores and you may re-infect yourself from your underclothes.

Use an acid gel (0.9% acetic acid in a jelly base available over the counter) to help maintain vaginal acidity so that Candida cells remain in their simple non-invasive form.

Take probiotic supplements and/or use a probiotic vaginal pessary.

Ask your partner to use an anti-fungal cream as Candida spores can survive under the male foreskin without causing problems. They may then be passed back to you.

If vulvovaginal symptoms are recurrent, have a vaginal health check at your local genito-urinary medicine clinic.

Candida And The Intestinal Tract

Candida yeasts are present in the gut of around 80% of healthy adults. When swabs are taken from apparently healthy volunteers, Candida can be grown from:

- the mouth of 1 in 2
- the oesophagus (gullet) of 1 in 10
- the rectum of 1 in 3
- the faeces of 8 out of 10.

In fact, it's likely that everyone has Candida growing in their gut at some time during every year, if not permanently.

Candida yeasts enter your gut through your mouth, mostly from food and drink but also from the skin of your hand when eating food or licking your fingers, by sucking items like pencils/pens or (in the case of babies) teats or nipples that have yeast cells on them. It's also possible to acquire intestinal yeast infections through kissing and oral sex.

Live Candida yeasts are found in a range of common foods, of which the worst culprits are fruit juices, ice cubes, salads, snacks and cereals. All vegetables and fruit can carry them, as yeasts are present on their skin when growing. Contamination of the final product is related to the type of packaging and processing used during preparation rather than the type of fruit involved. One study found that all juices sealed with foil wraps were contaminated, while those in cans or bottles were yeast-free.

Contamination of soft drinks dispensed in fast food restaurants and convenience stores, and unfinished drinks that are put aside for a while then sipped from again, directly from the bottle, is also common.

Candida And The Mouth

Your teeth chew and grind food into small pieces to help moisten them with saliva. Saliva contains enzymes (eg amylase) which start breaking down fats and starchy carbohydrates (into simpler sugars) within the mouth. The moistened food is then rolled into a small ball (bolus) by the tongue and pushed to the back of your mouth where it is swallowed in a reflex action. Yeast cells present in your food easily survive this process.

Oral Candida infections can occur at any age, but are seen most often in babies up to the age of 18 months, and in older adults aged over 65 years.

Yeasts prefer some sites in the mouth more than others, and in order of preference these are the upper surface of your tongue, your palate and the inner surfaces of your cheeks.

Oral thrush, and other mouth infections, are more common if you smoke or have:
- gum disease (gingivitis, periodontitis)
- a dry mouth (xerostomia) with poor saliva production due to increasing age, health problems (eg Sjogren's syndrome, following head radiotherapy), taking certain drugs (eg some antihistamines) or prolonged mouth breathing
- asthma or chronic obstructive pulmonary disease and use inhaled corticosteroids to control the underlying inflammation (a good inhaler technique and rinsing after use helps to prevent Candida)
- diabetes, especially if you also smoke which lowers your resistance to oral thrush even more
- impaired immunity through use of broad-spectrum antibiotics, illnesses such as leukaemia, other cancers or HIV or AIDS. In people with HIV, oral thrush is more likely to develop if your CD4 cell count drops below 350.

People who wear dentures are especially prone to oral thrush, in which case infection is referred to as denture stomatitis. Candida yeasts can stick to denture material which then act as a continuous source of reinfection.

The symptoms of oral thrush may include all or some of the following:
• a thick, white-yellow coating on the tongue
• a red, sore, shiny tongue
• sores at the corners of the lips (angular stomatitis)
• white plaques inside the cheeks
• soreness or itching eg on roof of mouth, beneath dentures
• pain on eating or drinking
• ulceration inside the mouth.

When oral thrush forms cream-white, curd-like plaques in the mouth the infection is diagnosed as acute (recent onset) pseudomembranous (false-membrane) candidiasis. This can persist for months in people using inhaled corticosteroids, chemotherapy or broad-spectrum antibiotics. The plaques are easily rubbed away and contain yeast cells, hyphae (germ tubes), inflammatory cells, bacteria, lining cells from the mouth, food debris and dead cells that are starting to break down. Underneath the plaque is a raw, tender area that is usually painful, red and may bleed.

When the plaques are dislodged (eg through eating) they leave behind a shiny, red, glossy area that is referred to as acute (recent onset), erythematous (red), atrophic (wasted) candidiasis. On the tongue, these areas are usually associated with a local loss of taste buds. If left untreated, the lesions take on a lumpy, granular appearance as underlying cells and blood vessels multiply in an attempt to heal small areas of ulceration. This is referred to as chronic (long-term) atrophic (wasted) candidiasis.

If undiagnosed and untreated, these areas can thicken and develop tough, white membranes with a roughened surface. These tend to be larger than the false membranes seen in early thrush infections and cannot easily be scraped away or dislodged during eating. This stage of oral thrush is known as chronic (long-term) hyperplastic (thickened) candidiasis, or candidal leukoplakia (white patches). It is important that this type of white patch is biopsied and properly diagnosed. Other conditions - some of which are precancerous - also cause white patches (leukoplakia) in the mouth and these need to be picked up early and treated to prevent mouth cancer. This is an excellent reason to attend for regular dental check-ups!

Investigation

Oral thrush is usually diagnosed by looking in the mouth and seeing characteristic areas of redness and white patches. Swabs can be examined under the microscope for yeast cells, hyphae and spores, or sent for culture in the laboratory to confirm the diagnosis and rule out other causes of leukoplakia.

Treatment

Mild infections may respond to a hexetidine antiseptic mouthwash or gargle used 2 or 3 times a day. Otherwise, recent onset oral thrush is easily treated with antifungal gels (eg miconazole, see Chapter 4). NB If you are pregnant or breast feeding, don't use any preparations before checking with a pharmacist or doctor:

If your mouth is really sore, a local anaesthetic spray (eg benzocaine) or anti-inflammatory spray/rinse (eg benzydamine) will help to numb the pain.

If you have oral thrush and use dentures, cleanse them thoroughly and apply a miconazole oral gel to the fitting surface before insertion (for short periods only). Leave dentures out at night, and for as often as possible during treatment. If the problem doesn't settle down, and swabs confirm that Candida is present, new dentures may be needed. If swabs are negative, another problem such as friction, bacterial infection or even allergy may be the cause.

Persistent oral thrush may need treatment with oral antifungal drugs on prescription.

Prevention

A mouth wash containing chlorhexidine has some anti-Candida action and may help to keep recurrent oral thrush at bay - but check with your dentist first. Not all dentists recommend chlorhexidine mouthwashes, and they can stain your teeth with prolonged use.

If you suffer from a dry mouth, an artificial saliva spray will help to keep your mouth moist and discourage infection. Sucking sugar-free pastilles containing malic acid also stimulates saliva flow

If you wear dentures, it is important to keep these scrupulously clean and not let stains build up. Keep them in a sterilising solution at night and have them checked regularly by your dentist for signs of wear or infection, and to check their fit.

Most people with asthma need to use a corticosteroid inhaler regularly to damp down the inflammation in their lungs. Even when inhaled correctly, up to 90% of the medication will deposited in the upper airways and then swallowed - only around 10% of the dose reaches the lungs. As the corticosteroid works by damping down excessive immune reactions in the tissues it touches, this makes oral thrush more likely. Rinse your mouth, clean your teeth or use a mouthwash or gargle immediately after using your inhaler (especially if it is a dry powder inhaler) to remove remaining particles. If recurrent oral thrush is a problem, ask your doctor about using a device such as a spacer to help minimise the amount of drug that is deposited in your throat.

People with gum disease are four times more likely to develop a thrush infection than other people. If you have redness or swelling of the gums round your teeth, or if your gums bleed when brushing or when you wake, you have gingivitis (infected gums). This harbours bacteria and yeasts in infected pockets between your gums and teeth. If ignored, infection can spread to involve the

46

jawbone round your teeth (periodontitis) and your gums will start to recede. Ignore periodontitis and you will eventually lose your teeth altogether.

Unfortunately, twice daily cleaning of teeth is not enough to solve gum disease. What you need is an expert assessment of your mouth with a dentist committed to oral hygiene, followed by a course of treatment with a dental hygienist. By having your gum pockets cleared of infected plaque and rotting food, gum disease can be beaten. You will then need to continue with a regular programme of proper brushing and flossing to keep your mouth healthy and disease free.

Sores at the corners of the mouth where the lips meet (angular stomatitis) is sometimes a sign of iron deficiency anaemia. If you feel tired and washed out, or if the problem is recurrent, ask your doctor if you need a check for anaemia.

If you smoke, do your utmost to stop. Smoking damages the lining of your mouth, lowers immunity, increases the risk of oral thrush and is also linked with mouth cancer.

Mouth cancer

Mouth cancer is becoming increasingly common. While it is not especially linked with Candida infection, it can be triggered by long term infections (sepsis) of the mouth, ill-fitting infected dentures, or may be mistaken for chronic hyperplastic candidiasis (see previously).

Mouth cancers usually start as a whitish patch (leukoplakia) or a red velvety patch (erythroplakia), both of which can mimic Candida infections. These pre-cancerous changes may cause a slight burning sensation in the mouth, but most are painless. As the tumour develops, it forms a small, raised lump which eventually ulcerates or forms a deep crack. This may bleed as it spreads into surrounding tissues and may then become painful.

Early diagnosis and treatment of an oral cancer leads to a cure in three out of four cases. Sadly, the outlook is poor if a mouth cancer has grown large before it is picked up. Those that develop on the roof of the mouth or top of the tongue may be spotted early, but those on the floor of the mouth, under the tongue or in coffin corner - an aptly nick-named crevice lurking at the back of your throat - are difficult to detect in the early stages. This is one reason why regular dental check-ups are advised.

Always seek medical advice about a mouth lesion that does not respond to anti-thrush treatment within two weeks.

Candida And The Oesophagus

Candida can be grown from the oesophagus (the tube connecting the mouth and stomach) of one in ten healthy people, but is usually present as a harmless commensal kept in check by the continual flushing action of eating, drinking and swallowing that wash Candida cells down into the stomach.

When active infection occurs because of an underlying problem with the immune system or an abnormality of the oesophagus itself, the lower two thirds of the oesophagus, nearest the stomach, are most usually affected. This may be a result of underlying damage previously caused by acid refluxing up from the stomach into the gullet. One in two people with Candidal overgrowth in the oesophagus also have oral thrush.

Candida infection of the oesophagus is more likely if you suffer from heartburn (gastro-oesophageal reflux disease) or any condition that interferes with normal swallowing such as:
- blockage of the oesophagus (eg scarring, thyroid goitre, tissue webs, tumour)
- pouching of the oesophagus (eg diverticulae)
- hardening of tissues (eg systemic sclerosis)
- nerve or muscle disorders (eg myasthenia gravis, motor neurone disease)
- poor muscular contraction of the oesophagus (achalasia).

Severe Candida infection of the oesophagus is usually associated with reduced immunity from a malignancy (eg leukaemia), drug treatment (eg chemotherapy, oral steroids, drugs used after transplant surgery) or acquired immune deficiency syndrome (AIDS). These conditions reduce the ability of immune cells (especially neutrophils) to limit Candida infection. In people living with HIV, oesophageal candidiasis is most likely to develop if your CD4 cell count falls to 200 or less. In these cases, oesophageal Candia infection is considered an AIDS-defining illness. This means that when HIV-infected patients develop oesophageal candidiasis, their condition has progressed to AIDS. Antiviral and antifungal drugs can significantly improve your health, however, and treatment advances are continuing to improve the outlook.

Candida overgrowth of the oesophagus may cause no symptoms, or may result in:
- difficulty swallowing
- pain on swallowing
- pain behind the breastbone
- nausea or vomiting
- bringing up blood (haematemesis)
- fever.

If left untreated, the raw areas may heal on their own but this can lead to scarring and narrowing of the oesophagus, with recurrent swallowing difficulties. If you notice any symptoms that you think may be due to infection, ulceration or narrowing of the gullet, tell your doctor without delay. These symptoms should be taken seriously to diagnose the underlying cause.

Investigation and treatment

If you develop problems with swallowing, or if Candida infection is suspected, you will most likely have an endoscopy so a doctor can visualise your throat and oesophagus directly. This involves light sedation with an injection (eg diazepam) into a vein on the back of your hand. Your oesophagus is then examined with a narrow, flexible endoscope containing a light, a camera and a tiny biopsy device. The doctor can directly view the walls of your oesophagus to identify any abnormal areas such as ulcers, strictures or Candida plaques. If a Candida fungal infection is found, it can be graded according to its severity:

Grade 1: scattered raised white plaques up to 2mm in diameter
Grade 2: numerous plaques larger than 2mm in diameter
Grade 3: plaques that merge together to form long white patches or nodules with some ulceration
Grade 4: as grade 3, but with swelling and narrowing of the oesophagus and easy bleeding on touching the walls.

During endoscopy, the doctor will take small biopsies for examination under the microscope. Infected areas of the oesophagus can also be swabbed for culture and microscopy. This gives direct evidence of invasion of tissues by a yeast infection. Brushings are more accurate than biopsies alone - in one study, 100% of brushings taken from the oesophagus were positive for Candida, compared with only 16% of biopsies on the same patients.

Treatment of oesophageal Candida is with antifungal drugs (See Chapter 4).

Prevention

The risk of Candida infection of the oesophagus can be minimised by avoiding heartburn and preventing acid damage to tissues in the lower oesophagus. One of the commonest causes of heartburn is acid reflux, in which stomach contents reflux up into the oesophagus. This damages and inflames the tissues lining your lower oesophagus and makes Candida infection and overgrowth more likely.

Normally, acid reflux is prevented by a muscle sphincter between the oesophagus and upper stomach, and by downward contractions (peristalsis) of muscles in the wall of the oesophagus. These protective mechanisms may fail due to poor muscle co-ordination, weakness of the stomach sphincter, the presence of a hiatus hernia, or increased pressure on the stomach from excess weight or eating too much.

Acid reflux causes a hot, burning sensations in the chest that may rise up into the throat. It usually comes on within 30 minutes of eating a meal and may be triggered by eating too much, taking exercise, bending or lying down. Meals containing fat, pastry, chocolate, acidic fruit juices, coffee or alcohol are the commonest culprits. There are several self-help measures that will help to control symptoms:

- Lose any excess weight
- Avoid smoking cigarettes
- Eat little and often throughout the day, rather than having three large meals

- Drink fluids little and often, rather than large quantities at a time
- Avoid hot, acid, spicy, fatty foods
- Avoid tea, coffee and acidic fruit juices
- Cut right back on alcohol intake - preferably avoid it altogether
- Avoid aspirin and related drugs (eg ibuprofen)
- Avoid stooping, bending or lying down after eating
- Avoid late-night eating
- Elevate the head of the bed about 15-20 cm (eg put books under the top two legs)
- Wear lose clothing, especially around the waist.

If symptoms of heartburn last more than a week or two, or keep coming back, consult your doctor and tell him or her what remedies you have already tried. Your symptoms may need investigation. Research suggests that 1 in 10 people taking regular antacids - especially those over the age of 40 - could have a more serious underlying problem such as a stomach cancer - which is easier to treat successfully if detected at an early stage .

Candida And The Stomach

Food usually spends around six hours in your stomach where it is churned by muscular contractions and mixed with powerful secretions containing hydrochloric acid and digestive enzymes. These break down proteins, fats and carbohydrates into simpler units to produce a porridge-like slurry known as chyme. The pyloric sphincter at the exit from the stomach then opens for a few seconds at a time to squirt chyme through into the first part of your small intestines.

After the oesophagus, the stomach is the most common site where active Candida infection can occur within the intestinal tract. Candida yeasts stop growing once acidity falls to a pH of 4.5, so at normal levels of acidity they are only present in small numbers as a harmless commensal. If immunity is reduced, or stomach acidity drops significantly, yeast cells can survive to pass further down the gut, or to cause a localised infection.

Glands in your stomach lining normally produce around three litres of acidic fluid per day. Production of stomach acid decreases with age, and the mucus lining the stomach wall also becomes thicker and stickier, coating any yeast cells present and further protecting them from the acid that is produced. This problem is compounded if antacids are also taken to treat heartburn, indigestion or peptic ulcer symptoms.

Candida can be grown from one in three biopsies taken from stomach peptic ulcers, and infection should be suspected in anyone whose stomach ulcer doesn't heal with usual treatment - especially in the elderly. In one study, five out of seven elderly patients with stomach ulcers that did not improve with standard antacid drugs healed within a month of adding antifungal medication.

Many people with active Candida infection of the stomach have no symptoms, while others develop non-specific problems that can include:

- loss of appetite
- weight loss
- early feelings of fullness after eating very little
- burning indigestion (gastritis) especially triggered by certain foods
- nausea or vomiting
- bringing up blood (haematemesis)
- abdominal pain
- fever.

If you develop any of these symptoms, tell your doctor as soon as possible.

Investigation and treatment

Stomach problems are usually investigated by endoscopy. A flexible instrument (gastroscope) is passed through the mouth into the stomach under light sedation. This allows direct examination of the inner walls of the stomach and the upper duodenum to visualise any inflammation, bleeding, ulceration or tumour. The procedure will also help to identify a hiatus hernia. Biopsies are taken from any suspicious-looking areas and examined under a microscope.

Candida infection of the stomach is treated with antifungal drugs (See Chapter 4).

Prevention

The risk of Candida infection of the stomach can be minimised by reducing factors that promote indigestion or which inflame the stomach lining (gastritis).

The terms *indigestion* and *dyspepsia* cover a variety of symptoms linked with eating, including sensations of burning and discomfort felt centrally in the upper abdomen.

Gastritis produces symptoms similar to those of a stomach ulcer, with burning or gnawing pain in the upper abdomen, nausea and vomiting. If gastritis is severe, you may even vomit and bring up blood-stained fluids (haematemesis). As the blood is usually partly digested, it is clotted and dark, resembling dark brown tea leaves or coffee grounds. Acute gastritis can be triggered by anything that irritates the stomach lining such as smoking cigarettes, excessive alcohol, aspirin, ibuprofen and other anti-inflammatory pain-killers known as NSAIDs (non-steroidal anti-inflammatory drugs) used to treat musculoskeletal problems such as arthritis or sports injuries.

The main cause of gastritis, however, is infection of the stomach with a bacterium called *Helicobacter pylori*. In the UK, at least 20% of 30 year old adults and 50% of those over 50 are infected. In some parts of the world up to 90% of adults are infected.

Helicobacter pylori is a mobile bacterium that burrows into the mucous lining of the stomach, leaving a breach through which acid can follow. Helicobacter also secretes an enzyme, urease, that helps to coat it with a small bubble of alkaline ammonia gas. This keeps the bacteria safe from acid attack but irritates the stomach wall leading to more inflammation. Infection can also let Candida yeasts penetrate through to the gut wall to set up an infection if your immunity is low.

Helicobacter pylori is linked with 85% of stomach ulcers and virtually all peptic ulcers in the first part of the small intestines (duodenum). One in three peptic ulcers are infected with Candida yeasts.

Helicobacter pylori is diagnosed through blood tests for antibodies to the bacteria, breath tests to detect urease activity, faecal antigen tests or from stomach biopsies taken during endoscopy. Once diagnosed, Helicobacter can be eradicated by triple therapy in which a combination of antibiotics and antacids are taken for 10 to 14 days.

> **Did you know?** *Research from New Zealand suggests that Manuka honey contains a unique antibiotic that can eradicate Helicobacter. Taking four teaspoons of Manuka honey, four times per day, on an empty stomach for eight weeks can wipe out a mild infection. If following an anti-Candida regime however, you may wish to avoid taking honey. NB If you suffer from diabetes, consult your doctor before using a honey treatment.*

To reduce the risk of gastritis or a stomach ulcer:
- stop smoking
- avoid alcohol which can cause chemical irritation of the stomach (gastritis)
- reduce your intake of tea and coffee

- avoid aspirin and related drugs such as ibuprofen
- eat several small meals per day rather than three larger ones
- avoid stress and take regular rest and relaxation
- follow a relatively bland diet and avoid foods that are acidic, hot or spicy.

Candida And The Small Intestines

The small intestines form a highly coiled tube around 285cm long, and 3.5cm across. The first part of the small intestines is the duodenum. Intestinal juices secreted into the duodenum are alkaline to neutralise the acidity of contents newly arriving from the stomach. Bile from the liver and powerful enzymes from the pancreas also flow into the duodenum to start the next phase of digestion.

The jejunum is the name given to the first 40% of the small intestines below the duodenum, while the next 60% is known as the ileum. There is no distinct border between the two and this division is somewhat arbitrary. Surprisingly Candida cells can survive quite happily throughout the small intestines, becoming more and more frequent as they get closer to the large intestines.

As food travels through, it is mixed with intestinal juices (succus entericus) secreted by glands in the small intestines lining. Of the 7 litres of fluid secreted per day, most is reabsorbed so that only 1-2 litres pass through into the large bowel.

Normally, the contents of the first part of the small bowel, the duodenum and upper jejunum, are virtually sterile due to the powerful digestive enzymes flowing in from the pancreas, and because the porridge-like chyme squirted through from the stomach flushes bacteria and yeasts further down the intestinal tract. Despite this, Candida yeasts can be isolated from the duodenal secretions of one in 25 healthy volunteers (sampled using a naso-gastric tube) and from the jejunum of one in two apparently normal, healthy adults.

Yeasts and bacteria can survive passage through the stomach to reach the small intestines (duodenum, jejunum, ileum) if:

- stomach acidity is reduced by antacids
- stomach acidity is reduced in later life
- yeast cells are coated and protected by the extra-sticky mucus produced in older people
- your stomach empties more quickly than usual (eg due to gastro-enteritis or irritable bowel syndrome)
- a large quantity of yeast cells is ingested
- a peptic ulcer acts as a reservoir of infection.

As samples are taken lower and lower down the small intestines, the likelihood of culturing Candida yeasts increases. This implies that yeast cells can survive exposure to strong alkaline chemicals and enzymes that join the duodenum from the bile and pancreas. The fact that Candida can survive in concentrated bile is no longer in doubt, since yeasts are grown from up to 2% of gall-bladders removed surgically.

The inner lining of the small intestines is covered in tiny projections ,around 1mm long, called villi. These increase the surface area of the intestinal wall to speed up absorption of the products of digestion, including amino acids, fats, sugars, vitamins, minerals and fluid. The villi also provide a large surface area on which yeast cells can stick and thrive without being washed away.

The binding sites used by Candida yeasts are also used by other microorganisms such as Lactobacilli. These 'friendly' bacteria also secrete substances that interfere with yeast growth and, together with the antibodies (type IgA) secreted onto the inner surface of the gut, help to prevent this reservoir of potential yeast infection from over-growing.

Most people with Candida overgrowth of the small intestines have taken broad-spectrum antibiotics, suffer from malnutrition or a serious illness that depletes their Lactobacilli population to lower their natural intestinal defences. This is not always the case, however, and a number of otherwise well people develop symptoms linked with Candida overgrowth in the small intestine.

In one study, fifty adults with recurrent diarrhoea and a variety of gastro-intestinal symptoms had a heavy growth of *Candida albicans* in their stool. In another case report study, six patients with small bowel candidiasis, five of whom had no obvious underlying illness or immune problem, and only two of whom had recently taken antibiotics. Their main symptom was diarrhoea that lasted from four days to three months. Once they started a course of anti-fungal treatment (oral nystatin), their symptoms disappeared within three to four days.

Babies with diarrhoea may also have a Candida infection of the small intestines. When 96 newborn babies with oral thrush were investigated, all were found to have Candida in their faeces, and 33 had diarrhoea with strands of actively growing yeast colonies (hyphae and mycelium) in their loose bowel motions. All got better with antifungal treatment. Six other babies developed diarrhoea but only had simple yeast cells in their stools; there were no signs of Candida activation or overgrowth and these did not respond to antifungal drugs. It is thought that diarrhoea in these babies may have been due to an allergic reaction to the yeast cells rather than to an active infection (See Candida Hypersensitivity Syndrome). Another study involving 24 babies with diarrhoea and positive stool cultures for Candida reported that all got better within one to eight days of starting anti-Candida treatment (nystatin).

Symptoms

In most cases, the presence of Candida cells in the small intestines is harmless. If it over grows and invades the wall of the small intestines however, it can produce symptoms such as:

- sensitivity to certain foods
- flatulence and bloating
- nausea and even vomiting of bile-stained fluids

61

- abdominal pain
- diarrhoea - which is usually watery, explosive and intermittent
- ulceration of the intestinal wall leading to bleeding.

Candida And The Gallbladder

Your gallbladder is a pear-shaped pouch beneath the liver in your upper right abdomen. It measures around eight by four centimetres and its sole function is to store bile and to intermittently contract and relax, releasing bile. These contractions become progressively stronger during a meal as food is churned within your stomach. During the night, and during other periods of fasting, the gallbladder still contracts strongly ever few hours in response to nerve signals and an intestinal hormone, called motilin (which also triggers intestinal contractions to move bowel contents onwards). As a result, your gallbladder regularly empties 20% to 30% of its stored bile even between meal.

Bile acid salts have a strong suppressive effect on *Candida albicans* to stop growth. This 'fungistatic' action is seen with all bile salts, but especially with cholic acid (sodium cholate) which causes Candida cells to swell. It also stops Candida yeasts from sticking to the lining of the gut so they are more readily flushed away. These actions all depend on having a healthy gallbladder and biliary tract, good immune function, and normal bile production, however. If bile production is reduced or your gallbladder contracts poorly, Candida yeasts may manage to colonise the gallbladder or, especially if the biliary tract is compromised by invasive procedures such as endoscopic retrograde cholangiopancreatography (ERCP) or immune function is significantly reduced (eg by intensive chemotherapy). Candida infection of the gallbladder (fungal cholecystitis) will lead to symptoms of vomiting, fever and abdominal pain.

Although considered relatively rare in healthy people, a study published in the journal of Gastrointestinal Endoscopy in 2009 stated that infection of the biliary tract with Candida and other fungal species has increased in the last few years. They looked at 123 patients undergoing a procedure known as ERCP (see below) in Germany and found Candida species in bile samples from 54 (44%). Biliary candidiasis was only suspected in seven of these patients before the yeast was identified, however. Biliary candidiasis was not associated with positive mouth or stool cultures (so routine swabs are unhelpful in diagnosing the problem). In this study, Candida infection was strongly associated with having reduced immunity (eg progressive cancer, chemotherapy, severe illness requiring intensive care) and with taking long-term antibiotics. Although surgical contamination could not be totally excluded, the researchers felt this was unlikely. When they repeated the study in 2014, Candida species were detected in bile samples from 38 out of another 127 patients. The yeasts were identified as mainly *Candida albicans* (60%) or *Candida glabrata* (16%) and rarely as *Candida parapsilosis*, *Candida tropicalis*, or mixed species.

Candida And The Large Intestines

By the time food reaches the end of the small intestines and passes into the large bowel, the process of digestion is complete and most nutrients absorbed. The large intestines are mainly concerned with taking up excess fluid, salts and minerals from the remaining bowel contents. From around two litres of semi-liquid contents arriving in the large bowel each day, 90% of the fluid is absorbed so that only 200 - 250 ml of semi-solid waste remains for voiding.

The large bowel forms a wide tube that is around one metre long and consists of the colon, rectum and anal canal. The large intestines are home to billions of bacteria that ferment indigestible fibre waste reaching the colon to produce acids and gases, as well as many useful vitamins such as biotin. Bowel micro-organisms - including yeasts - make up around 30% of normal stool bulk. The colon is therefore the main site in which yeast cells can thrive in the normal gut, although normally they are present in the harmless form. Ten species account for over 97% of the fungal population found in the gut, of which *Candida albicans* and *Candida parapsilosis* are the most common.

> **Did you know?** *The appendix is a blind-ending pouch branching from the first part of the colon (caecum). The appendix averages 10cm in length, but can vary between 2cm and 22cm. Because of its long, thin shape it is referred to as the vermiform (worm-like) appendix, or vermix. Although it is often viewed as a vestigial organ left over from ancient times, it contains lymphoid tissue and may play a role in gut immunity. It also acts as a reservoir for healthy digestive bacteria (lactobacilli) to replenish the gut after taking antibiotics, or after a vomiting and diarrhoea illness (gastroenteritis). However, people who have their appendix removed do not seem to come to any harm as a result. It's possible that the appendix acts as a reservoir for Candida yeast infection, too.*

The lining of the large bowel (mucosa) is different from that in the small intestines. It does not contain absorption villi and is richly supplied with glands that secrete a lubricating mucus. Mucus production is mainly stimulated by the mechanical contact of faeces with the colon wall.

The three muscle layers of the large bowel are arranged in a different way to those in the stomach and small intestines. The outer layer of muscle fibres are collected together into three longitudinal bands (called Taenia coli). Because these bands are shorter than the rest of the colon, they act rather like drawstrings that draw the wall into out-pouchings known as haustra. These pouches provide an ideal hiding place for bacteria and yeasts to grow and multiply.

Bowel bacteria are usually beneficial, in that they:
- ferment and help to break down undigested fibre
- provide bulk to make defecation easier
- compete with potentially harmful bacteria and yeasts for nutrients which helps to suppress their overgrowth
- make acids and natural antibiotics/antifungal substances that inhibit growth of other organisms
- make and secrete vitamin K, B group vitamins, biotin and folic acid which can be absorbed and used in the body
- absorb some cholesterol and fatty acids from the gut preventing their reabsorption - when some antibiotics are given, blood cholesterol levels (especially the more harmful LDL-cholesterol) can rise.

Did you know? Over half the weight of your stools consists of bacteria.

Candida yeasts can be grown from rectal swabs in 30% of healthy people who have no symptoms of ill health - the yeast cells are present as harmless commensals. If conditions in the large bowel change to favour Candida overgrowth however (such as following a prolonged course of antibiotics) symptoms such as bloating, loose stools and flatulence may develop. Once these problems arise, Candida can be grown from stools of as many as eight out of 10 sufferers.

Symptoms

Symptoms of Candida infection of the large intestines include:

66

- sensitivity to certain foods
- flatulence
- bloating
- watery diarrhoea, usually without blood or excess mucus
- constipation
- uncomfortable spasm and straining when trying to pass a stool (tenesmus)
- other symptoms consistent with irritable bowel syndrome.

Some researchers feel that diarrhoea is also triggered in some people without an overgrowth of Candida, when an allergic reaction is triggered against Candida products (See Candida Hypersensitivity Syndrome).

Investigations and treatment

The investigation of large bowel symptoms usually involves an abdominal and a digital rectal examination. Stools may be cultured to look for bacteria, parasites or Candida, although if yeasts cells are found, they may not be reported if they are in their simple cell form (no hyphae) as they are assumed to be a normal part of the bowel flora. You may also have tests for hidden blood (faecal occult blood) and, if necessary, an ultrasound to check for thickening of the bowel wall, tumours or anatomical abnormalities.

The lining of the lower bowel can be examined via sigmoidoscopy (insertion of a telescope fitted with a light and camera to examine the lower, sigmoid colon) or colonoscopy (insertion of a longer, more flexible instrument to inspect further up the colon, usually under sedation). You will be given a powerful laxative to take beforehand which acts within 10-14 hours. This empties the bowel to provide a better view.

Candida And Inflammatory Bowel Diseases

Inflammatory bowel diseases (IBD), as the name suggests, are associated with inflammation of the digestive tract.

Crohn's disease is a chronic, relapsing and remitting condition in which the full thickness of the intestinal wall becomes thickened, fissured, ulcerated and inflamed. The end of the small intestine (terminal ileum) is frequently involved, but it can affect any part of the gut from the mouth to the anus. Typically, discrete 'skip lesions' are seen, with apparently normal bowel between inflamed regions. Crohn's disease can come on at any time, but most often appears during adolescence and early adulthood. Males and females are equally affected.

Ulcerative colitis is a long-term (chronic), relapsing and remitting inflammatory disease that affects just the inner lining (mucosa) rather than the full thickness of the bowel wall, and develops in the rectum and a variable length of the colon. It is twice as common as Crohn's disease, and affects around one in 1000 people, but the prevalence varies widely from country to country.

Ulcerative colitis and Crohn's disease appear to be two different conditions, but they are not well understood and sometimes it is impossible to determine exactly which condition is present. These cases are diagnosed as 'indeterminate colitis'.

What are the symptoms?

The symptoms of inflammatory bowel disease include passing blood-stained diarrhoea which may also contain pus and mucus. In severe attacks fever, abdominal pain, fatigue and feeling unwell also occur. Attacks tend to come on every few months although some people have infrequent symptoms, and for others they are continuous. Both conditions are linked with inflammation elsewhere in the body such as the joints (arthritis), eyes (iritis) and skin (eg erythema nodosum).

What are the causes?

Inflammatory bowel diseases are believed to result from an interaction between the environment, genetic and infectious factors. The genetic associations are stronger in Crohn's disease than in ulcerative colitis. An autoimmune attack is thought to be triggered against an unidentified colonic bacterium, virus or other parasite initially, then a cross reaction attacks the large bowel lining in susceptible people. Abnormal bowel fermentation or poor blood supply to the gut wall may also be involved.

One of the latest findings is that a sugar 'force field' is activated within the bowel lining when your defences are down. This encourages the growth of protective probiotic bacteria so they are able to suppress the over-colonization of harmful micro-organisms such as Candida. If the gene (IL-22RA1) needed to make this protective shield during times of stress is faulty, intestinal cells cannot produce more sugars, protective bacteria are not stimulated, and inflammatory bowel disease is more likely to develop.

What is the treatment?

Medical treatment includes drugs that reduce inflammation such as aminosalicylates and corticosteroids (oral or topical enemas and foams). In severe Crohn's disease, antibody treatments (eg infliximab, adalimumab) aimed against a particular immune marker (TNF alpha) are used to reduce inflammation. Antibiotics may be prescribed, but until recently, antifungal treatments were not tried.

The role of Candida in inflammatory bowel disease

Candida yeasts are commonly found in the intestines of people with inflammatory bowel disease (IBD), but whether they are a contributing cause, or taking opportunistic advantage to invade an already damaged gut wall remains unclear. Whichever is the case, their presence is likely to provoke inflammation, increase symptom severity and delay healing.

Until recently, most microbiologists focussed on gut bacteria when investigating inflammatory bowel disease, but now attention is turning towards yeasts. This is because of a recognition that inflammatory bowel disease and gastrointestinal Candida colonization are both associated with raised levels of a signalling chemical (a cytokine called IL-17) which is produced by immune cells and may underlie the ability of Candida yeasts to enhance inflammation.

Candida and ulcerative colitis

People with ulcerative colitis are frequently colonised by Candida species and, in those with active disease, treatment with the antifungal drug, fluconazole, led to a reduction in clinical signs and in the size of inflammatory lesions to reduce their disease severity. A number of studies have now confirmed that the presence of *Candida albicans* delays healing of ulcerative colitis lesions.

Clinical scientists investigating the role of intestinal fungi believe they have identified a key immune receptor abnormality that may be involved in persistent Candidiasis in some people with ulcerative colitis. This receptor, Dectin-1, is found on intestinal lining cells. It is also present on macrophages (immune scavenging cells) and allows them to recognise and attack any fungi that try to breach the gut wall. Mice that are Dectin-1 deficient have an increased susceptibility to inflammatory bowel disease, and treating them with antifungal drugs helps to reduce the severity of the disease. By comparing the Dectin-1 gene between humans with severe ulcerative colitis and those with less severe symptoms, researchers from King's College, London, have identified a particular mutation that might predict which patients with ulcerative colitis will develop more severe disease, and might also benefit from antifungal treatment. Dectin-1 is also acting as a focus for developing future drugs.

Diet and ulcerative colitis

Researchers have compared the food and drinks consumed by people with ulcerative colitis to the visual appearance of the bowel lining and pinpointed the dietary components most likely to trigger active symptoms as follows:

Foods linked with active ulcerative colitis
Burgers, sausages and other preserved meats (except organic, non sulfited products)
Beer (except German beer, which is sulfite free), lager
Red and white wine
Sulfite-containing soft drinks eg fruit squash made from concentrates
Coffee (except de-caffeinated brands)
Prawns, scampi, shellfish (sulfited)
Dried fruit and vegetables (sulfited)
Processed fruit pies and fruit cakes
Foods containing sulfites (check labels)
Foods containing the sulfur-rich seaweed, carrageenan (Irish Moss, E407)

Foods containing sulfites (added as a preservative) or caffeine are particularly important triggers. Some sulfur compounds (eg hydrogen sulfide) have been shown to damage the bowel lining and produce changes similar to those seen in ulcerative colitis. Although the bowel is usually able to detoxify these sulfur substances, this ability may be reduced in people with ulcerative colitis as higher than normal bowel levels of sulfur compounds are detectable.

However, no foods consistently provoke symptoms in all people, so it's important to keep a food diary to help pinpoint the foods that provoke your own attacks. Some people are sensitive to dairy and wheat produce, for example, and find it helpful to follow a gluten-free diet. Others are more likely to relapse after a high intake of red and processed meat, protein and alcohol.

Some varieties of probiotic bacteria (especially Lactobacillus and Bifidobacter species) have shown benefits in preventing relapses and maintaining remission. Probiotic bacteria produce butyrate, a short-chain fatty acid that provides energy for bowel lining cells (colonocytes). Abnormal metabolism of butyrate has been suggested as a possible cause of ulcerative colitis, and probiotic bacteria help to maintain butyrate levels. They may also work, of course, by suppressing the presence of Candida yeasts in the gut.

Candida and Crohn's disease

Researchers from Tufts University, Boston, studied patients with Crohn's disease and their unaffected, healthy relatives, as well as healthy controls living in the same area. They found an association between familial Crohn's disease and *Candida albicans* colonisation, with relatives of people with Crohn's also showing increased leakiness of the gut and increased likelihood of Candida colonisation, even though they were Crohn's-free. One theory is that Crohn's develops when, for some reason, normal interactions between intestinal micro-organisms and host defences break down. Although the trigger remains unknown, analysis of a large database of patient records identified a statistically significant link between antibiotic use – especially with tetracyclines – and the subsequent diagnosis of Crohn's disease.

French researchers have also found that 80% of the yeast cell wall is made up of substances called glycans, and that in people with Crohn's disease, antiglycan antibodies are often present, establishing a previously unsuspected link between Crohn's and *Candida albicans*. Others have found that people with Crohn's disease have low levels of defensins, natural antibiotics secreted by intestinal cells to kill Candida and other potential infections. These lower levels may explain why Candida is able to take hold. And, in an interesting experience, live white blood cells (neutrophils) from people with Crohn's disease and from healthy volunteers were incubated with Candida cells to see what would happen. After 30 and 60 minutes, the white cells from the controls had killed significantly more Candida cells, suggesting that neutrophils from people with Crohn's disease have an impaired ability to kill them.

> ***Did you know?*** *People with inflammatory bowel disease often have low levels of riboflavin (B2), folate, beta-carotene, vitamin B12, calcium, phosphorus, magnesium, selenium, zinc and vitamin D. A multivitamin and mineral supplement will help to reduce nutritional deficiencies.*

Diet and Crohn's disease

Researchers have developed the so-called LOFFLEX (low-fibre, fat-limited exclusion) diet to treat Crohn's disease. This excludes foods that have been identified by bowel specialists as most likely to worsen symptoms. It limits fat intake to around 50g per day, and fibre to 10g, and should be followed under the supervision of a medical nutritionist or dietician.

Foods that are NOT allowed
Pork
Fish in batter/oil/tomato
Milk (cows, goat, sheep) and dairy products
Wheat, rye, barley, millet, buckwheat, corn, oats
Yeast
Pulses, onion, tomatoes, sweetcorn
Citrus fruit, apples, bananas, dried fruits
Vegetable, corn and nut oils
Nuts and seeds
Tea, coffee, alcohol, squashes, cola

After following the LOFFLEX approach for two weeks, new 'test' foods are introduced, one at a time, every four days, as long as you remain symptom free. Wheat products must be tested for seven days, as the onset of symptoms is often delayed after its reintroduction. If a test food causes side effects, continue to avoid it and wait until all symptoms have improved before testing another food. If no reactions occur, you start testing a new food after four days.

> **Did you know?** *In one study, over half of people who followed the LOFFLEX diet were still free from symptoms after two years.*

Probiotic supplements promote a healthy balance of intestinal bacteria. Some probiotic strains have been shown to prevent relapses of Crohn's disease symptoms, and to help maintain remission.

Candida And Irritable Bowel Syndrome

While overgrowth of Candida in the gut produces ulceration and inflammation which can be diagnosed and treated, the presence of non-invasive Candida in the bowel is now also thought to trigger symptoms of diarrhoea-predominant irritable bowel syndrome in some people. This may be linked with an allergic hypersensitivity reaction against Candida yeasts.

Irritable bowel syndrome (IBS) is a problem of bowel function rather than structure and is linked with abnormal or exaggerated bowel movements and muscular spasm. It is the most common condition to affect the gut, and at least a third of the population are affected at some time during their life, even if only mildly. Overall, 15% of people are affected badly enough to consult their doctor.

In order to diagnose irritable bowel syndrome there must be (in the absence of other causes) recurrent abdominal pain or discomfort for at least three days per month in the last three months, associated with two or more of the following:

- Improvement with defecation
- Onset associated with a change in frequency of stools
- Onset associated with a change in form (appearance) of stools

These diagnostic pointers are known as the Rome III criteria and, although symptoms should have followed this pattern for the last three months, they should have started 6 months prior to diagnosis.

While a diagnosis of IBS should ideally occur after other potential causes of the symptoms have been ruled out, the label is often applied with no attempt to exclude other conditions such as Candida (or even bowel cancer). So-called 'Red Flag' factors that suggest something else is causing the symptoms, such as an inflammatory bowel disease or bowel cancer, include:

- Rectal bleeding
- Iron-deficient anaemia
- Weight loss
- Fever
- Onset after 40 years of age
- Family history of colon cancer
- Nocturnal symptoms
- Faecal soilage.

If any of the above red flags occur, seek medical advice as soon as possible.

Many people with IBS develop symptoms for the first time after an attack of food poisoning (gastroenteritis) or taking antibiotics. Both factors disrupt the normal balance of bacteria found in the bowel, affect the normal process of fermentation in the colon and change the amount and composition of bowel gases produced.

During 1994, 38 victims of an outbreak of Salmonella were studied by researchers and, over the next year, almost a third (12 out of 38 or 32%) went on to develop recurrent bowel symptoms consistent with IBS. In most cases, they developed intermittent diarrhoea. Those with the worst symptoms (diarrhoea lasting more than seven days plus vomiting leading to weight loss) were more likely to develop IBS than those with milder infective symptoms. They also took longer to recover their appetite, weight and energy levels.

Another study looked at 75 patients admitted to hospital with bacterial gastroenteritis. Of these, 22 (29%) had symptoms three months later that were consistent with IBS. Nine out of ten of these were still suffering after six months and three quarters still had IBS problems one year later. Again, those with the worst symptoms (diarrhoea lasting longer, with abdominal pain and mucus in the stools) were more likely to develop IBS.

Researchers are unclear why bacterial bowel infections are linked with IBS, but a sensitivity to Candida products, or to a yeast overgrowth which somehow interferes with normal bowel function have been suggested.

Taking a probiotic supplement during and after a course of antibiotics helps to replenish levels of 'friendly' bowel bacteria and may help to limit Candida overgrowth.

Is Candida involved in IBS?

Patients with diarrhoea-predominant IBS often have intermittent, persistent, watery diarrhoea, accompanied by gas distension, flatulence and abdominal pain. These are also the main symptoms caused by intestinal Candida infection. However, a link between the two has proved elusive and, if Candida is diagnosed, this obviously rules out IBS by definition (it should only be diagnosed in the absence of other recognised causes).

A case-controlled study from Addenbrooke's Hospital, Cambridge, was published in 1992. Stool samples were cultured from 38 patients with IBS and 20 healthy controls. Moderate numbers of *Candida albicans* (10,000 per gram) were grown from three of the stool samples provided by IBS patients (7.9%) but from none of the controls. These findings were dismissed as two patients had recently received antibiotics and one stool sample was delayed in transit by more than 24 hours. When these individuals were resampled, no Candida colonies were grown. The authors therefore concluded that C. albicans was not a cause of irritable bowel syndrome.

Despite the above, it is known that certain proteins in the wall of *Candida albicans* yeasts (mannans, mannoproteins) and secreted candidal enzymes (aspartyl proteinases, enolase) can trigger allergic responses, heighten reactions against other allergens (eg the egg protein, ovalbumin) and can provoke mast cell-mediate 'leakiness' of the intestinal lining. In fact, an astounding 178 different antigens (proteins that can trigger an allergic reaction) have been identified in Candida species. This may explain the high number of cross-reactions experienced when eating foods containing other yeasts and moulds.

A paper published in the European Journal of Gastroenterology and Hepatology in 2005 accepted that, although the role of yeasts in IBS remains unclear, there is increasing evidence that yeasts can cause IBS-like symptoms in sensitive patients as a result of the antigenic proteins and enzymes they produce. This might explain why symptoms can worsen after eating mould-containing foods. The authors added that much of this work is controversial, and that more research is needed before antifungal treatments can be recommended as a first-line treatment for IBS. Sadly, in the ten years since that paper was published, researchers appear to have steered clear of this topic and there are no further findings to report.

Candida And Lactose Intolerance

A test for deficiency of the enzyme, lactase, will identify whether or not Candida-like bowel symptoms are due to lactose intolerance.

Lactose is a sugar, found in milk, which must be broken down during digestion into two simpler sugars (glucose and galactose) before it can be absorbed. This is achieved by lactase enzyme which is produced by the lining of the intestine during infancy. After weaning, lactase enzyme production falls and, if you produce insufficient amounts, lactose sugar remains undigested and unabsorbed. It passes through your small intestines to reach the large bowel where it is fermented by bacteria and Candida yeasts to produce typical symptoms of bloating, diarrhoea and cramps.

Inability to digest lactose sugar is a fact of life for much of the world's adult population. In Asia, lactose intolerance is almost universal after infancy. It affects over 75% of people with Afro-Caribbean genes and half of people living in South America. North-western Europeans and those with European ancestry (such as white North Americans) are likely to produce lactase into adulthood but 15% of adults in these populations, on average, are lactose intolerant.

Investigation and treatment

Lactose deficiency can be confirmed by medical tests, but simply cutting out milk products for two weeks will show whether or not symptoms improve. If symptoms worsen again when re-introducing milk, then lactose intolerance is likely.

Hydrogen breath test: After drinking a lactose solution, the breath is analysed for hydrogen at regular intervals. If hydrogen breath levels increase over time, it suggests that bacteria are fermenting undigested lactose in the intestines.

Blood glucose test: After drinking a lactose solution, blood samples are taken at regular intervals. If blood glucose levels do not rise, it suggests that lactose is not being broken down by lactase (to form glucose and galactose).

Stool acidity test: Fermentation of undigested lactose by gut bacteria produces lactic acid which is expelled in the stools. Increased stool acidity can indicate lactose intolerance.

Treatment of lactose intolerance essentially means avoiding all products that contain lactose. This isn't as simple as switching from cows' milk to goat's milk or sheep' milk as these contain similar levels of lactose. Low lactose cows' milk, cheese, yogurts and cream are available, however (eg Lactofree range). The lactose content of different milks is as follows:

Milk source	Lactose (g) per glass
Full fat cows' milk	9.3 g
Skimmed cows' milk	9.8 g
Low lactose cows' milk	Less than 0.5 g

Goats' milk	8.6 g
Sheep' milk	9.9 g
Soy milk,	0
Rice milk	0
Oat milk	0
Nut milks	0
Coconut milk	0

> *Did you know?* cows' milk yoghurt has a low lactose content as bacterial fermentation breaks down lactose. Many people with lactase deficiency can tolerate yogurt, fromage frais and aged cheese.

Lactose lurks within milk derivatives such as whey, whey sugar, hydrolysed whey and caseinate salts such as sodium caseinate. It is commonly found in

- Bread and cereals
- Tinned soups
- Ice cream
- Processed meats and ready meals
- Salad dressings
- Cakes
- Cream liqueurs
- Non-aged cheeses (eg cottage cheese)
- Pill coatings.

> *Did you know?* Some medicines contain lactose – ask your pharmacist if those you are taking are lactose-free.

Taking a digestive enzyme supplement containing lactase may enable you to continue to eat and enjoy lactose-containing products if you wish.

Candida, Gluten And Wheat Intolerance

If bowel symptoms come on after eating wheat products and improve when you eliminate these from your diet, you may have a wheat protein intolerance. If your symptoms dramatically improve on avoiding wheat and other grains, you could have undiagnosed gluten intolerance. Sensitivity to wheat gluten can come on at any age and affects up to one in 100 people, yet for everyone who knows they have gluten intolerance – a condition known as coeliac disease - another seven remain undiagnosed. It is more common in females than males and often runs in families.

What is gluten?

Glutens are the proteins that give bread dough its elasticity and are found in several cereals including wheat, rye, barley and oats.

Wheat gluten contains a small protein chain (peptide) called gliadin which can trigger an immune reaction in some people. Those sensitive to wheat gluten are often sensitive to the glutens found in other cereals, too, because of the similar peptides they contain. In fact, it is relatively common for people with coeliac disease to react to rye and barley, but they are less likely to react to the gluten in oats. Maize usually causes no problem.

Grain	Form of gluten
Wheat	gliadins
Rye	secalins
Barley	hordeins
Oats	avenins
Maize	zeins

In coeliac disease, the presence of gluten in the gut causes sensitised immune T-cells to attack the lining of the small intestine. Antibodies aimed against the intestinal lining (anti-endomysial antibodies) are also produced against tissues (endomysium) within the jejunal wall. Normally, the jejunal lining is covered in tiny projections around 1mm long, called villi, which increase the surface area of the intestinal wall to speed absorption of nutrients. In people with coeliac disease, eating gluten causes the villi to disappear so the lining of the jejunum becomes abnormally smooth. As a result, the absorption of nutrients is reduced. These changes are reversible when gluten is excluded from the diet.

> **Did you know?** *Half of people with coeliac disease have anaemia due to poor iron or folic acid absorption. Consider taking a multivitamin and mineral supplement aimed at your age group – but ask your doctor if you need a blood test to check for anaemia first.*

What are the symptoms of gluten sensitivity?

Symptoms of gluten intolerance vary in severity and may come on suddenly or creep up over months or years. At one end of the spectrum is coeliac disease which is associated with:

- Increasing tiredness
- Abdominal pain, bloating and wind
- Diarrhoea or vomiting
- Passing pale, bulky, offensive, fatty stools that float
- Weight loss if gluten is not excluded from the diet.

At the other end of the spectrum is non-coeliac gluten sensitivity (NCGS) involves parts of the body other than the gut and is even more common and insidious. This type affects between 7% and 35% of the population, depending on how it is defined. Typical symptoms can include:

- Feeling tired all the time, or chronic fatigue
- Generalised feelings of being unwell
- Breathlessness or asthma
- Joint inflammation and pain
- Skin changes such as pigmentation, scaliness, eczema and other rashes.

Skin symptoms tend not to develop in people with the abdominal symptoms of coeliac disease, although everyone is different.

Is Candida involved in gluten sensitivity?

What triggers gluten sensitivity is unknown, but one theory is that exposure to a particular virus (eg rotavirus, Adenovirus 12) might stimulate the production of autoantibodies in people who have inherited certain genes. It is more common in those with other autoimmune conditions such as type 1 diabetes, ulcerative colitis or autoimmune thyroid disease.

In 2003, a paper published in The Lancet proposed that *Candida albicans* might act as a trigger for the onset of coeliac disease. A virulence factor secreted by some yeasts, called hyphal wall protein-1 (HWP1) contains several amino acid sequences that are highly similar to those in alpha-gliadin and gamma-gliadin. HWP1 is used by *Candida albicans* to stick to the intestinal wall. Although the theory is complicated, they suggest that the combination of a yeast bound to certain components of the intestinal lining (tissue transglutaminase, endomysium) might stimulate the formation of anti-endomysial antibodies aimed against both HWP1 and gluten which could then cross-react with the jejunal lining. Candida yeasts might, therefore, lead to wheat intolerance or even trigger coeliac disease in genetically susceptible people.

Intolerance to other proteins found in wheat (not gliadin) can also cause symptoms that may be misdiagnosed as intestinal Candida or as irritable bowel syndrome. Although not classed as coeliac disease (as no anti-endomysial antibodies are present), following a wheat-free diet will significantly improve symptoms.

Little is known about the cause of non-coeliac gluten sensitivity, but one theory suggests that symptoms result from poor function of mitochondria - the tiny cell organelles that produce energy in all cells, but especially muscle cells, which might explain the lack of energy and persistent fatigue.

> ***Did you know?*** *Co-enzyme Q10 supplements can boost energy production in mitochondria and may reduce persistent fatigue. Usual doses are 100mg (ubiquinol form) to 200mg per day (ubiquinone form) but higher doses may be suggested by a medical nutritionist in some cases.*

How is coeliac disease diagnosed?

If you think your Candida-like symptoms may be due to gluten sensitivity, your doctor can arrange a blood test to look for the presence of anti-endomysial antibodies.

Following a gluten free diet

If coeliac disease is confirmed, you will need to follow a gluten-free diet for life – this will allow your intestinal villi to redevelop and your symptoms to disappear.

A gluten-free diet allows you to eat a wide variety of foods, including:
• Fruit, vegetables, and salad stuff including potatoes
• Beans, peas, lentils
• Nuts and seeds
• Fresh or frozen unprocessed meat, poultry or offal
• Plain (uncoated) fish
• Eggs, cheese, milk, yoghurts (except muesli yoghurt)

- Soya bran, rice bran, rice, tapioca, sago, arrowroot, buckwheat (which despite its name is not related to wheat), millet, hempseed, teff, maize, corn and cornflour
- Gluten-free bread, crispbread, biscuits, cakes, breakfast cereals and pasta
- Gluten-free flour, soya flour, potato flour, pea flour, rice flour, gram flour
- Sugar, jam, marmalade, honey, jelly
- Herbs, spices, mustard, vinegar, salt, pepper
- Milk, cream, butter, margarine and oils
- Tea, coffee, fruit juice
- Wine, non-barley beer, spirits.

Check food labels carefully for hidden gluten as wheat is often present in products such as soups, stock-cubes and dessert mixes. Avoid any foods labelled as containing Wheat, Gluten, Gliadin, Flour starch, Wheat flour, Wheat starch, Food starch, Edible starch, Modified starch, Gelitinised starch, Vegetable starch, Cereal filler, Cereal binder, Cereal protein, Malt, Rye, Hydrolysed vegetable protein, Kamut, Natural flavouring, Soy Sauce, Gum, Triticale, Spelt, Rusk, Barley unless they are declared gluten-free (wheat can be processed to render it gluten-free).

> *Did you know?* *Some medicines contain gluten – ask your pharmacist if those you are taking are gluten-free. Gluten is also added to some cosmetic products but rarely listed in the ingredients. Although gluten is not absorbed through the skin, when used in lipstick or foundation small amounts can be ingested. If bowel or skin symptoms persist, despite a gluten-free diet, try using cosmetics labelled as gluten-free to see if this helps.*

If you have coeliac disease and eat foods containing gluten, your symptoms will recur, although some people may find they tolerate small amounts. Gluten free versions of cereal-containing foods such as bread and cakes are widely available. In the UK, you can obtain some gluten-free staple foods on prescription from your doctor. For more information visit www.coeliac.org.uk.

If you have gluten-intolerance without anti-endomysial antibodies, a digestive enzyme supplement containing gluten protease, cellulase and amylase may help.

Systemic Candida

The most serious type of Candida infection is systemic candidiasis, in which yeast cells spread throughout the body to infect two or more organs such as the liver, kidneys, lungs, heart, spleen or brain. This only usually occurs where there is a major breakdown in immune defences such as when:

- A large number of yeast cells are present that swamp the immune system
- The normal bacterial content of the gut is disrupted leading to massive Candida overgrowth (eg after a prolonged course of antibiotics)
- The immune system is suppressed (eg with immunosuppressive drugs or a serious illness such as leukaemia, lymphoma or AIDS)

- The lining of the gut is severely damaged (eg severe ulceration or trauma).

Candida yeasts mainly enter the body from the intestines. This is known as translocation. When only a small number of yeast cells are involved, these are quickly mopped up by macrophage scavenger cells or neutrophil pus cells unless the immune system is suppressed. When large numbers of Candida are present, however, even someone with a healthy immune system may become seriously ill. This was proven historically by a medical doctor who drank a solution containing one billion Candida yeast cells. He developed signs of sepsis (fever and shakes) within three hours. Yeast cells were found in his bloodstream and urine within six hours.

Modern research suggests that live yeast cells can move across the bowel lining into the blood stream and lymphatic system from all parts of the digestive system, but mainly from the jejunum in the small intestines. Blood from the intestines contains absorbed nutrients and travels straight to the liver, so this is usually the first organ to show signs of a systemic Candida infection (eg small abscesses), closely followed by the spleen which filters cells and infections from the blood.

Candida yeast cells can also cross into the circulation from the lungs, but this is thought to account for only one in thirty systemic Candida infections.

Systemic candidosis is a real threat in hospitals as in-patients often have illnesses or treatments that weaken their immune defences. Among hospital acquired infections seen in intensive care units, Candida infection is number four on the list of culprits. In the United States, out of around 80,000 blood infections treated each year, 11.5% were due to Candida yeasts. Of these, half were due to *Candida albicans*, while the others involved closely related species such as *Candida glabrata* and *Candida krusei*. Another study found that up to 20% of infections involving medical implants such as central venous lines, bladder catheters and artificial heart valves were due to *Candida albicans*.

Once Candida infection is suspected or confirmed by blood cultures, treatment is with high-strength antifungal drugs, usually given by intravenous injection initially.

Candida Hypersensitivity Syndrome

Many people have inexplicable, non-specific and recurrent symptoms that are difficult to treat. These frequently include:

- Fatigue or tiredness all the time
- Irritability, anxiety or depression
- Difficulty concentrating and sleeping
- Headache, joint and muscle pains
- Sugar and carbohydrate cravings
- Recurrent cystitis with no evidence of bacterial infection
- Irritable bowel-like symptoms

- Alcohol intolerance
- Premenstrual aggravation of symptoms in women.

In some cases, these symptoms come on, or worsen, after taking broad-spectrum antibiotics, raising the suspicion that Candida is to blame. However, culture tests are usually negative and anti-fungal treatments do not seem to help.

As far back as 1990, a trial was conducted to see whether antifungal treatment was effective in Candida hypersensitivity syndrome. The study involved 42 premenopausal women with fatigue, premenstrual syndrome, intestinal symptoms and a history of recurrent Candida vulvovaginitis. During the 32-week trial, each woman received four different combinations of the antifungal drug, nystatin, or placebo (inactive treatment). These were used either orally or vaginally, so that each women used each regime (oral and vaginal nystatin; oral nystatin and vaginal placebo; oral placebo and vaginal nystatin or all-placebo) in eight-week blocks. Neither they nor the researchers knew which tablets or pessaries were the active ones until the code was broken at the end of the trial.

As expected, the three active-treatment regimes including nystatin were more effective than placebo in relieving vaginal symptoms. However, the nystatin did not reduce the systemic symptoms significantly more than placebo. On average, the scores for systemic symptoms (eg fatigue, premenstrual syndrome) improved by 25% when using one of the three active-treatments and by 23%

with the all-placebo regime. The researchers concluded that, in women with presumed candidiasis hypersensitivity syndrome, nystatin does not reduce systemic or psychological symptoms significantly more than placebo and that long-term nystatin therapy is not indicated.

It was then suggested that these symptoms could have been triggered by the presence of a yeast infection that, although long disappeared, left its mark in the form of an immune over-reaction to Candida proteins. For example, Candida proteins absorbed into the circulation might interact with immune cells to trigger a response against the presence of low numbers of commensal, non-invasive yeasts in the gut. Although the theory behind Candida hypersensitivity syndrome is controversial, it is accepted that when antibodies bind to circulating foreign proteins (antigens) to form soluble complexes, symptoms such as fatigue and feeling non-specifically unwell (malaise) usually result.

Another possibility is that the normal presence of Candida yeast cells living relatively harmlessly in the gut makes the intestinal lining more leaky. This would allow incompletely digested food particles to enter the circulation more easily. Once this leakiness has occurred, the immune system may become sensitised to these food particles to produce a variety of non-specific food intolerance symptoms. This would explain why anti-fungal drugs do not improve the problem.

At present, the use of antifungal drugs in Candida hypersensitivity syndrome is only advised when the presence of yeast infection is proven. Oral drugs have potential side effects and are unlikely to help, or may make problems worse (and contribute to drug resistance) when used inappropriately. However, some people find that taking antifungal supplements and/or following an anti-Candida diet is helpful.

Where recurrent diarrhoea is linked with hypersensitivity to yeast cells on skin testing (usually performed by a private practitioner or dermatologist) and where Candida are cultured from bowel motions, bowel symptoms have been shown to get worse when given Candida extracts to eat. In these cases, antifungal treatment to eradicate bowel Candida, and following an anti-Candida diet may help.

CHAPTER 2

Nutritional Approaches

Candida sensitivity and overgrowth can be overcome through diet and lifestyle, but it is important to avoid fad diets and over-strict regimes that are difficult to follow, make life a misery and can lead to vitamin and mineral deficiencies. Many people are advised by well-meaning nutritionist to cut out all fruit, limit vegetables, eat almost no grains and to avoid all the foods that give pleasure in life in order to 'starve' the yeasts of sugar and carbohydrates. Paradoxically, these diets often make things worse and lead to deteriorating health and reduced immunity that actually promote persistent Candida overgrowth.

Laboratory research shows that *Candida albicans* grows quite happily in the relatively low concentrations of glucose (100mg/dl equivalent to 5.5mmol/l) found in normal blood and tissues, so trying to starve yeasts of sugar in the intestines is not going to prevent its survival. In fact, immunologists now know that when you are under stress, your intestinal lining cells actually produce extra sugar to promote the growth of healthy, probiotic bacteria, to

97

help keep Candida at bay. So, starving yourself of healthy sugar sources may have adverse effects against your protective intestinal microbes. The best anti-Candida diet is one that boosts immunity rather than one that deprives you of adequate nutrition. The modern functional medicine approach to Candida and intestinal leakiness involves what is known as the 5 Rs approach which stands for:

Remove (eg parasites, food intolerances)

Reintroduce (eg proper chewing, dietary fibre, vitamins and minerals, sufficient stomach acidity, digestive enzymes and bile)

Re-inoculate (friendly digestive bacteria)

Repair (eg with vitamin D, omega-3s, l-glutamine, Aloe vera and curcumin)

Re-balance (your diet and lifestyle).

Some of the vitamin, mineral and herbal supplements mentioned here are discussed in more detail in the next chapter which also gives the doses. This overview is designed to explain the benefits of each step and why it is undertaken.

Remove

The Remove phase of the 5Rs approach involves eliminating unwanted factors such as parasites and the foods to which you are intolerant.

Remove parasites

When indicated (for example by recurrent diarrhoea) stools are sent for culture to look for potential parasites such as *Blastocystis hominis*, *Dientamoeba fragilis*, *Entamoeba coli*, *Endolimax nana* and *Giardia lamblia*. All but Giardia are often found as commensals in the intestines of healthy people without symptoms, however, and their presence is therefore often discounted. If found in someone with persistent problems, antibiotics may be prescribed to aid their eradication. Natural anti-parasitic treatments that may be suggested by a nutritional therapist or naturopath include curcumin, Echinacea, garlic, grapefruit seed, olive leaf, oregano oil and sage extracts.

Remove food intolerances

Food intolerance is a reproducible, adverse reaction to a specific food or ingredient which occurs even when that food is eaten in a disguised form. These reactions tend to come on slowly and may be delayed for hours or even days after eating the trigger food, making it difficult to identify the culprits.

Food intolerance is not the same as a classic food allergy, which involves a type of antibody called immunoglobulin E (IgE). Ig E is believed to have evolved to protect against certain gut parasites such as Schistosoma worms. In some people with an allergic tendency, IgE is triggered against other foreign proteins such as those found in certain pollens, venoms or foods such as peanuts. When these foreign proteins are encountered, IgE is released as a signal to activate the immune system and serious, life-threatening reactions can occur such as swelling of the face, difficulty breathing, low blood pressure and collapse (anaphylactic shock). These symptoms come on rapidly, usually within minutes of contact with the allergen.

In contrast, the symptoms of food intolerance are not linked with IgE production, and tend to come on more slowly after exposure to the trigger and are unpleasant but not life threatening.

Non-IgE mediated food intolerances are divided into four broad categories:
- Pharmacological (drug-like) reactions to chemicals present in food such as histamine (eg scombroid fish such as tuna, tomato, fermented foods, cheese, spinach, aubergine, berries, citrus); Monosodium glutamate (Chinese restaurant syndrome); Tyramine (eg cheese, wine, yeast extract, vinegar); Sulphites (mainly in people with asthma); Tartrazine and other artificial colours; Preservatives (eg benzoates, sorbates, nitrates, nitrites).
- Enzyme deficiencies such as lactose intolerance.
- Autoimmune reactions such as gluten intolerance.

100

• Food-specific IgG antibody reactions which, although controversial, can be used as a test to look for Candida sensitivity.

The majority of your immune cells actually reside in the lining of your small intestines, in what is known as GALT (gut-associated lymphoid tissue). This is both diffusely distributed and, within the ileum, are concentrated into nodules known as Peyer's patches. Peyer's patches contain specialised M-cells that constantly sample fluids within the intestines, taking tiny 'sips' which they transport into the centre of the patch for inspection. Here, immune cells (T and B lymphocytes) may generate a response, including the production of antigen-specific antibodies as a first-line defence against any infection present in the gut.

M-cells are highly selective. They only transport antigens (protein fragments capable of triggering an immune response) that bind to molecules on their surface. This helps to avoid activating the immune system against innocuous food antigens. Foreign proteins can evade this selective immune processing, however, by passing between the gut lining cells though normally 'tight' junctions if these become 'leaky'. A leaky gut is associated with factors such as immaturity (eg in infants under the age of 12 months), drinking alcohol (which dehydrates the junctions and doubles the rate of allergen uptake), infection (eg Candida), inflammation, physical exertion and other forms of stress. For example, someone who does not usually react against shellfish may do so after eating a seafood risotto, washed down with wine at a beachside café, then climbing up a steep cliff path in the heat of summer. This combination of

101

factors can compromise the integrity of a normally 'tight' intestinal lining.

When food is digested, the proteins it contains are broken down into their basic building blocks – amino acids - before they are absorbed into the circulation. Single amino acids do not trigger an antibody response. If the gut is 'leaky' however, longer chains of amino acids (peptides) may be absorbed intact. Although controversial, this theory is supported by research in which egg yolk and cows' milk proteins have been found in human breast milk. The only logical way in which they could have got there is through the blood stream from the gut.

The immune system is designed to recognise and attack foreign proteins (antigens). This is usually achieved by scavenger cells and by producing a type of antibody (IgG) to mop them up.

Circulating IgG antibodies protect the body against viruses, bacteria and fungi. When they bind to an antigen, they activate scavenger cells and trigger the formation of complement 'protein bombs' which blow holes in the side of bacteria and yeasts. Levels of IgG antibodies aimed against certain infections are measured to assess immunity against, for example, measles, mumps, rubella and hepatitis B. The presence of high titres of IgG against a particular infection represents good immunity.

Low levels of anti-food IgG antibodies can be detected in the blood of most people, and do not usually cause problems as food antigen-

IgG complexes are removed by scavenger cells without triggering a cascading immune response. In some people, however, eating foods to which they have an elevated level of food specific IgG antibodies may cause symptoms during the following days. These symptoms tend to be non-specific and, although controversial, are thought to include:

- Tiredness and lack of energy
- Stuffed up, runny nose or excess mucus
- Headache or migraine
- Pre-menstrual syndrome
- Eczema, psoriasis and other skin problems, including acne and rosacea
- Asthma, wheezing or shortness of breath
- Joint aches and pains, including backache and 'rheumatism'
- Bloating, abdominal pain, diarrhoea and other symptoms that may be diagnosed as irritable bowel syndrome or Candida.

Although this field of research has not attracted much attention, studies have linked raised levels of IgG antibodies with cow's milk intolerance (anti-casein IgG), egg intolerance (antiovalbumin and anti-ovomuvoid IgG) and to migraine, asthma, adenoid enlargement, rheumatoid arthritis and irritable bowel syndrome (IBS).

People with IBS have found their symptoms significantly improve when eliminating the foods to which they have raised IgG levels. A study by the University of York investigated the effectiveness of a three month exclusion diet in 150 people with IBS and raised levels of specific anti-food IgG antibodies (based on the YorkTest FoodScan test). The double-blind, randomised, controlled trial showed that eliminating the identified foods provided significantly greater symptom relief than eliminating 'sham' foods to which participants were not intolerant. The researchers concluded that a clinically significant improvement was achieved in some patients with IBS using a food elimination diet based on IgG food antibodies.

IgG blood tests are expensive. As everyone has a different profile of foods which may trigger their symptoms, another way to find out if a nutritional approach will help you is to follow an elimination and challenge diet.

How to follow an elimination diet

The simplest type of elimination diet involves keeping a food and symptom diary for at least one week to help pinpoint potential culprit foods, and to avoid them until your symptoms settle. The suspect foods are then re-introduced, one at a time, every three or four days, to identify any that cause your symptoms to recur.

A more advanced approach involves following a bland, hypoallergenic, restriction diet that initially allows you to eat only a few limited items that most people tolerate, typically:

Grains: White rice, tapioca
Fruit: Pears, pear juice, cranberries

Vegetables: Squash, carrots, parsnips, lettuce, lentils, split peas
Meat: Lamb, wild game, turkey
Fluids: Spring, mineral or distilled water.

A strict elimination and challenge diet is best carried out under the supervision of a nutritional therapist. This approach is time consuming, can be difficult to stick to, and is nutritionally incomplete. Food-related symptoms tend to worsen on days Two to Four, improve by days Five to Seven, and usually disappear by days Ten to Fourteen. After symptoms disappear, you start re-introducing eliminated foods one by one, usually at three day intervals. During this time you keep a careful food and symptom diary to help identify problem foods. If your symptoms reoccur, you continue to avoid the test food and wait 48 hours after all symptoms have improved before testing another food.

When first re-introducing a food, you eat just a small quantity (eg 1oz cheese) at breakfast time and monitor for a recurrence of symptoms over the next four hours. If all is well, you eat twice the amount at lunchtime (eg 2 oz cheese) and again monitor for adverse reactions over four hours. If all is OK, you then eat twice as much again for dinner (eg 4 oz cheese). On the following day, you avoid the test food again and continue to monitor for delayed reactions. If there is no reaction, or results are unclear, you can reintroduce the test food again the next day in larger amounts. If you are certain you are not reacting to a particular food, it can become a normal part of your diet again, and you move on to testing another food. If you feel there is a definite link between your symptoms and eating a particular food, avoid it, then try it again at a later date to see if the effect is consistent.

Researchers have found that the people most likely to have a food sensitivity and who respond best to avoiding certain foods are those with diarrhoea. One study found that just under half of people with IBS-like symptoms (which are very similar to those associated with Candida) gained significant benefit from following an elimination diet. On average, each person reacted against two to five different foods.

- Avoiding milk products helped 50%
- Cutting out wheat helped 25%
- Eliminating citrus fruits helped 15%
- Avoiding coffee helped 10%.

If you do not want to follow a full elimination and challenge diet, you may find it helpful to cut out the most commonly troublesome foods (gluten, wheat, milk products, eggs, corn, coffee, citrus fruits, tea) until symptoms subside; then reintroduce them one at a time to see what happens. During this time, keep a careful food and symptom diary, recording:

- Everything you eat and drink and at what time
- Any symptoms
- What time symptoms start and how long they last
- Daily activities, stress levels and so on to look for patterns.

If your symptoms are not significantly improved by following a restricted diet, it is important to return to eating a normal diet, and to eating as wide a range of foods as possible, to guard against any nutrient deficiencies. If you are able to identify a small number of foods that undoubtedly provoke your symptoms however, these can usually be avoided without affecting your overall nutrition.

NB Do not follow a restricted diet long-term without seeking advice from a nutritionist or dietician.

Reintroduce

The Reintroduce phase of the 5Rs approach involves replacing any vital digestive components that are lacking, such as efficient chewing, sufficient fibre, vitamins and minerals plus the digestive enzymes, acidity and bile needed to process food properly. Any of these factors can be compromised as a result of diet, medication, certain diseases, the ageing process or hereditary factors.

Reintroduce proper chewing

Digestion starts in the mouth, where biting and chewing mechanically break down food ready for swallowing. While this may sound obvious, busy lifestyles and stress cause many people to bolt down their food before it is properly chewed. Mastication – the act of chewing – is vital not just to disrupt food but to moisten it with saliva. Saliva contains two digestive enzymes, amylase which splits starch into simpler carbohydrates such as maltose and glucose, plus salivary lipase which breaks down dietary fats.

Did you know? You produce between 750ml and 1500ml saliva per day while awake. Very little is produced during sleep. Salivary lipase is swallowed to build up in the stomach between meals - 20% of dietary fat is digested in the stomach by this enzyme.

If you chew food thoroughly, you are less likely to develop indigestion. You are also giving salivary enzymes more chance to attack any yeasts present in each mouthful. Naturopaths suggest chewing each mouthful twenty to thirty times, while stress experts suggest that you eat mindfully by focussing on each bite.

Mindful eating involves savouring and really experiencing the look, smell, texture and taste of each bite. Don't do anything else at the same time. Don't eat and read the newspaper, or eat and watch TV - focus solely on the food. To experience mindful eating, find a crisp, sweet, juicy apple and try the following exercise:

Sit comfortably, breathing slowly and deeply in a relaxed manner. Pick up the apple and note its colour, shape and texture. Inhale deeply so its complex scent fills your mind. Place the apple against your mouth and feel its waxy texture with your tongue. Now take a bite. Note the initial resistance and the way it 'gives' as your teeth cut through the crisp flesh. Feel the juice squirt into your mouth or dribble down your chin. As you chew, focus on the sounds that fill your head. Notice the sweet, fruity, sharp taste, and the texture of the flesh as it falls apart. Extract as much flavour as you can before swallowing each bite.

Reintroduce dietary fibre

Dietary fibre, or roughage, consists of the non-digestible carbohydrates in your diet. Even though fibre passes through your small intestines unchanged, and provides few nutrients, it is essential to:

- encourage secretion of intestinal juices
- aid the digestion of other foods
- slow the absorption of sugars and fats so your liver can handle them more easily
- promote the growth of beneficial bacteria
- cleanse the bowel
- promote bowel contractions
- absorb excess fluid and reduce looseness
- mop up toxins, yeasts and bacteria to aid their expulsion.

Together, these actions also discourage Candida overgrowth and can improve digestive symptoms in some people with diarrhoea or constipation, irritable bowel syndrome and other Candida-related symptoms.

> ***Did you know?*** *For every gram of fibre you eat, your bowel motions increase in weight by around five grams due to increased bacterial multiplication.*

All plant foods contain two types of fibre, soluble and insoluble, but some sources are richer in one type than another. Our ancestors' diet provided 100g or more fibre per day, but the modern diet often fails to provide the recommended intake of at least 20 to 30g daily.

Soluble fibre (eg pectins, gums) form a gel when mixed with liquid and are particularly important in the stomach and upper intestines, helping to optimise the digestion and absorption of sugars and fats.

Good sources of soluble fibre include oats, pearl barley, rye bread, figs, apricots, tomatoes, apples, courgettes, carrots, prunes, kidney beans and other legumes.

Once soluble fibre reaches your large bowel, it is fermented by bacterial enzymes to release nutrients (and smelly gas). The level of 'friendly' probiotic bacteria in the bowel is significantly improved by eating particular sources of fibre known as prebiotics. Supplements containing this type of fibre (eg fructo-oligosacchharides) are widely available.

Insoluble fibre (eg cellulose) is most important in the large bowel, where it adds bulk, absorbs water, bacteria and toxins, and hastens stool excretion. Good sources of insoluble fibre include bran, wheat, sweetcorn, brown rice, rhubarb, berries, leafy vegetables, peas, lentils, chickpeas. Supplements providing fibre that promotes bowel movements (eg bran, psyllium seed/ ispaghula) are also widely available.

When increasing your fibre intake, it is important to drink at least two to three litres of fluid per day to bulk up the fibre and prevent your motions becoming too dry. Many people who do not tolerate a high-fibre diet well are simply not drinking enough water.

NB Bran and phytates (found in unleavened wheat bread) bind minerals in the gut so they remain unabsorbed. This can reduce uptake of iron by as much as 65%, as well as reducing absorption of zinc, calcium and manganese. This problem does not occur with leavened (yeast-raised) bread, as yeast enzymes break down phytates so mineral-binding does not occur. However, high-fibre diets, which speed the passage of food through the bowels, will reduce the amount of minerals absorbed, especially calcium. If you are following a high-fibre diet, ensure you obtain enough calcium (eg from milk and dairy products, broccoli, nuts, seeds and pulses), iron, zinc and trace minerals.

Reintroduce any vitamins and minerals you are lacking

Although deficiency diseases linked to severe lack of vitamins and minerals are rare in the developed world, minor insufficiencies are common. National diet and nutritional surveys show that, although average intakes across a population may be OK, some people still do not obtain the lower reference nutrient intake (LRNI) below which deficiency diseases can occur. The micronutrients that are most often lacking are iron, magnesium, potassium, selenium and zinc. Vitamin D status also tends to be low during winter months. You cannot make vitamin D in your skin (from a cholesterol-like precursor) when the UV index is less than 3. All these micronutrients are important for immune function and your defences against Candida yeast overgrowth.

Iron is needed to make powerful chemicals used by white blood cells to kill invaders. Lack of iron alters the proliferation and activation of lymphocytes and natural killer (NK) cells, T-lymphocytes and scavenging macrophages. An important iron-binding protein, called lactoferrin, is present in body fluids and released from white blood cells (neutrophils) when they are fighting an infection. This lactoferrin clears iron from the tissues, acting as a first-line defence against invading organisms such as Candida which need iron to grow properly. A similar protein, called lactoferricin, also has a direct microbicidal activity against *Candida albicans*. Dietary sources of iron include shellfish, red meats, sardines, wheatgerm, wholemeal bread, egg yolk, green vegetables and dried fruit.

Magnesium is used as a co-factor by over 300 enzymes which cannot work properly when it is in short supply. It is involved in the production of T-lymphocyte cytokines – the chemicals that regulate the immune and inflammatory responses of other white blood cells. Lack of magnesium is believed to over-activate scavenger cells to increase inflammation, and also appears to hasten the programmed death of immune cells to shorten their lifespan. Women with recurrent Candida tend to have low magnesium levels, which also contributes to tiredness and fatigue. Dietary sources of magnesium include beans (especially soy), nuts, whole grains (although if these are processed they lose most of their magnesium content), seafood, and dark green, leafy vegetables. Chocolate, drinking water in hard-water areas, mineral seasoning salt and Brewer's yeast are also important sources.

Potassium levels are tightly regulated by the body to maintain a constant blood level. Its concentration inside cells is therefore thirty times greater than in the extracellular fluid. Inside immune cells, potassium is needed for the production of proteins and for the action of interleukin-1 beta – an important signal that triggers the initial

112

antifungal response. This trigger is now known to depend on potassium flooding out of the cell. Foods that contain potassium include seafood, fruit (particularly tomatoes, bananas), vegetables, whole grains and low-sodium potassium-enriched salts.

Selenium stimulates the production of natural killer cells which fight infections, and is also needed for antibody synthesis. Lack of selenium reduces the activity of T-lymphocytes and decreases antibody production. In the laboratory, immune cells from people lacking in selenium are significantly less able to kill Candida yeasts than those whose selenium levels are optimal. The best food sources of selenium are Brazil nuts, fish, poultry, meats (especially game), wholegrains, mushrooms, onions, garlic, broccoli and cabbage.

Zinc is needed for cell communication and the proliferation and activation of lymphocytes fighting infection. It interacts directly with the nucleus of immune cells, switching on genes to power up an attack against bacteria, viruses and yeasts. Lack of zinc is one of the main causes of reduced immunity seen in children with malnutrition, as it suppresses the thymus gland where T-lymphocytes develop and mature. Mild zinc deficiency is common in women with recurrent vaginal Candida. Zinc deficiency decreases resistant to Candida infection and reduces the ability of scavenger macrophages to absorb and destroy yeast cells. Dietary sources of zinc include red meat, seafood (especially oysters), offal, brewer's yeast, whole grains (although processing removes most of their mineral zinc), pulses, eggs and cheese.

113

Vitamin D regulates immune function through a direct interaction with the nucleus of immune cells to activate their response against bacterial, vial and yeast infections (for which zinc is also needed). This stimulates T-lymphocytes to regulate the immune response and increases antibody production within B-lymphocytes. The neutrophils (white blood cell scavengers) from people with an hereditary defect in vitamin D production have a 30% to 40% suppressed ability to kill *Candida albicans* compared to those with normal vitamin D levels. This effect may be linked to lower calcium levels.

> ***Did you know?*** *Vitamin D is a fat-soluble vitamin that occurs in five different forms, the most important of which are vitamin D2 (ergocalciferol) derived from plants, and vitamin D3 (cholecalciferol) derived from animals. These two forms are collectively known as calciferol. Food sources of vitamin D3 include oily fish, fish liver oils, animal liver, fortified margarine, eggs, butter and fortified milk.*

Biotin is a B vitamin that is widespread in the diet and produced by intestinal bacteria from which it is absorbed into the body. Deficiency is uncommon but an estimated one in 123 people has an inherited inborn error of biotin metabolism. This reduces the integrity of skin and mucus membrane linings so that yeast infection becomes more common. In such cases, high-dose biotin supplements will solve the problem.

Reintroduce sufficient acidity

The pH scale is a measure of the amount of acid (hydrogen ions) present in a solution, and ranges from 0 (highly acid) to 14 (highly alkaline). Pure water has a pH of 7 which is neutral. So, a pH value of less than 7 means a solution is acidic, while a value of greater than 7 shows a solution is alkaline.

The pH scale is logarithmic, which means that each 1 unit change in value represents a ten-fold change in hydrogen ion concentration. A solution of pH 4 is ten times more acidic than one of pH 5 and 100 times (10 times 10) more acidic than a solution of pH 6.

> **Did you know?** *Many carbonated soft drinks have a pH of 3, making them ten thousand times more acid than water (pH 7).*

Stomach juice normally has an acidity of around pH 2, but it can range from pH 1 to pH 3 between eating. When the stomach contains food and drink, the juices become more dilute and less acid, and the pH can rise to pH 4 to pH 5, which is still acidic but less so than normal.

Your stomach lining contains microscopic gastric pits containing glands that secrete mucous, digestive enzymes and two to three litres of hydrochloric acid each day. Secretion of hydrochloric acid is regulated by hormones, including gastrin which increases acid secretion, and somatostatin which inhibits its release.

Stomach acidity is designed to both break down food and to kill the microorganisms that are invariably present in food. Some microorganisms happily survive a short passage through stomach acid, especially the probiotic, acid-loving bacteria, Lactobacillus acidophilus and Candida yeasts. In very acidic conditions, Candida tends to stay in its less invasive form as simple yeast cells that occasionally bud and divide. When acidity falls below pH 4.5, Candida yeasts stop growing. As stomach acid is normally around pH 2, any yeasts present on or in the food and drink you consume are either killed or remain in the harmless, commensal form. As stomach juices become significantly less acid – for example if you take antacids – yeasts can thrive and, at pH 6 (just below neutral) may start to produce the invasive threads (germ tubes or hyphae) that trigger infection and symptoms. This switch from a simple-celled form to the thread form can occur within one to three hours of a loss of environmental acidity. As food tends to stay in the stomach for around four hours, on average, any contaminating Candida yeasts present may start to overgrow when acidity is reduced.

In people with lowered immunity, the stomach is one of the most common sites where active Candida infection occurs within the intestinal tract. This is because once food leaves the stomach and passes into the duodenum, it mixes with the bicarbonate-rich secretions of the small intestines and the environment chances to an alkaline one of around pH8 to pH9 which yeasts particularly dislike.

116

Poor stomach acid production promotes Candida growth and is relatively common. Hypochlorhydria means stomach juices are less acid than normal, while achlorhydria means stomach acid production has ceased.

Reduced stomach acidity can result from medication (eg proton pump inhibitors, h2-blockers), medical conditions including type 1 diabetes and gastritis (inflammation of the stomach) as well as following some types of gastric surgery, but often there is no obvious underlying trigger. Across Europe and the US, low stomach acid (hypochlorhydria) affects an estimated 15% of people. Very low stomach acid (achlorhydria) is seen in between 1% and 5% of otherwise healthy people and becomes more common as age increases. One study found that achlorhydria was present in just under 2% of people in their 50s, but in 19% of people in their eighties. Another study found reduced stomach acid levels in as many as 69% of elderly people.

> ***Did you know?*** *Lack of stomach acid reduces the absorption of minerals needed for healthy bones, including calcium, and increases the risk of hip fracture. It is also associated with reduced absorption of iron, leading to anaemia.*

Some people have reduced hydrochloric acid production as a result of producing antibodies aimed against their acid-producing parietal cells. These antibodies are found in as many as one in five people with type 1 diabetes and may also reduce the production of 'intrinsic factor' which is needed to absorb vitamin B12 lower down in the small intestines. Lack of B12 eventually leads to pernicious anaemia.

People with low stomach acidity may notice some of the following symptoms:

- Stomach ache, discomfort, bloating or burping after meals
- Feeling unwell/fatigue immediately after eating
- Food or water 'sitting' in the stomach
- Poor appetite or easily feeling over-full
- Nausea or stomach upset after eating high fat foods or supplements (eg fish oils)
- Difficulty digesting red meat
- The presence of undigested food in bowel motions
- Reflux and/or heartburn
- Constipation.

> *Did you know?* *Between 40% and 60% of people with asthma have low levels of hydrochloric acid, and this is twice as common in females with asthma than males. People with asthma also appear to secrete too few pancreatic digestive enzymes, are more likely to have gastroesophageal reflux disease, and to show abnormalities in the lining of their upper digestive tract. The reason is not fully understood, but researchers believe the reduced acid secretion is a cause, rather than a result of having asthma.*

If you think you may have low stomach acid production, seek medical advice.

A nutritional therapist may recommend taking cider vinegar (although this can contain yeasts), high dose vitamin C (ascorbic acid) or a digestive enzyme supplement containing betaine hydrochloride-pepsin (eg one capsule before each meal, slowly increasing to two, three or more if well tolerated). NB You will be advised not to use hydrochloric acid supplements with anti-inflammatory medications such as aspirin or ibuprofen as this , could increase the risk of peptic ulceration with bleeding or even perforation of the stomach.

Reintroduce sufficient digestive enzymes

An enzyme is a protein that triggers or speeds the rate at which a particular chemical reaction takes place. You produce 22 different digestive enzymes within your digestive tract. Those known as proteases (eg pepsin, trypsin) break down dietary proteins, amylases digest carbohydrates while lipases break down fats.

The level of digestive enzymes you produce depends on your genes, diet, lifestyle, gender and age. As you get older, you tend to produce less intestinal enzymes so your ability to absorb nutrients decreases. Lack of digestive enzymes has been linked with a number of health problems, from bloating, wind and heartburn to Candida, irritable bowel syndrome and rosacea.

> ***Did you know?*** *Digestive enzyme insufficiency can result from stress, nutrient deficiencies (especially lack of magnesium and zinc), smoking, high alcohol intake, overeating, low stomach acidity, and conditions such as pancreatic insufficiency, gallstones, coeliac and Crohn's disease, food allergies or intolerance and leaky gut syndrome.*

People with low stomach acidity may notice some of the following symptoms:
- Bloating after a meal and increasing throughout the day
- Excessive flatulence

- Diarrhoea-predominant irritable bowel syndrome
- Constipation
- Feeling full after eating only a few mouthfuls
- Sensation of food sitting like a 'stone' in your stomach
- Undigested food in your motions
- Stools that float and are unusually smelly.

Plant enzymes with a similar action to human digestive enzymes are found in fruit and vegetables, including cellulases that digest fibre. Eating a raw food diet will maximise your intake of active plant enzymes. When heated above 40 degrees Centigrade, these enzymes are denatured however, so cooked food contains little if any, natural enzyme activity.

Digestive enzyme supplements are available to treat a range of conditions, including those that promote the breakdown of Candida yeasts. These supplements are mainly derived from plants (eg pineapple, papaya, kiwi, fungi) but some are from animal sources (eg pancreatic enzymes from pigs). Plant enzymes are usually considered superior as they are more stable over a wider range of acidity, and are less likely to be broken down by stomach acids.

Digestive enzyme products often contain other ingredients that promote enzyme action such as betaine HCL (to boost the hydrochloric acid content of the stomach), extract of ox bile (an animal-derived enzyme that stimulates intestinal movements) and fructo-oligosaccharides which promote growth of probiotic bacteria in the bowel.

Enzyme products are generally selected according to symptoms that suggest intolerance to a particular food group (fats, proteins, and carbohydrates) or to particular foods (eg fruit, milk, yeast, gluten-containing cereals). If you feel bloated after eating carbohydrate, for example, select a product that contains carbohydrate-digesting enzymes such as amylase and cellulase. If milk causes a problem, consider a product containing milk-digesting enzymes such as bromelain (from pineapples), papain (from papaya), lipase and lactase. If you are gluten-intolerance, a product supplying gluten protease, cellulase and amylase can help.

If you want to improve general digestion or are not sure which food group is causing the problem, select a mixed digestive enzyme supplement containing lipase (digests fats), amylase (digests carbohydrates), protease (digests protein), lactase (digests milk sugar) and cellulase (digests cellulose).

Enzyme supplements designed to dissolve the cell wall of Candida yeasts typically contain a blend of some, or all, of the following: cellulase, hemicellulase, amylase, invertase and glucoamylase, protease, pectinase, Papain and Bromelain. It is usually best to seek advice from a nutritional therapist to ensure you take the most suitable enzyme mixture for your particular situation.

Dose: Normally 1 to 4 capsules – you may need to experiment to find the best dose to help your symptoms.

Check labels for 'activity units' as these show the potency of the enzymes present in a supplement. Those with the highest number of activity units are the most active.

Digestive enzymes are normally taken at the beginning of a meal to help improve digestion-related problems. To treat other problems such as Candida, you may be advised to take them on an empty stomach. If taking the enzymes for indigestion, don't take an antacid or indigestion remedy within two hours of taking the digestive enzymes as this may reduce the effectiveness of the enzymes.

If your symptoms do not improve within two weeks of taking digestive enzyme supplements, stop taking them and seek medical advice.

Reintroduce bile sufficiency

Bile acid salts have a strong suppressive effect on *Candida albicans* cells, so they stop growing. This 'fungistatic' action Is seen with all bile salts, but especially with cholic acid (in the form of sodium cholate) which causes Candida cells to swell. It also stops Candida yeasts from sticking to the lining of the gut so they are more readily flushed away. These actions depend on producing normal amounts of bile. If immune function is significantly reduced (eg by chemotherapy or taking long-term antibiotics), if bile production is reduced, or if the biliary tract is compromised (for example by surgery or invasive procedures such as endoscopic retrograde cholangiopancreatography – known as ERCP) then Candida yeasts can colonise the gallbladder. In some cases, this can lead to infection and inflammation (fungal cholecystitis) with vomiting, fever and pain, although this is relatively rare.

Bile is a green-yellow, bitter-tasting fluid that is made in your liver and trickles down into your gallbladder for storage until needed. When your gallbladder contracts, bile flows down into the first part of your small intestines (duodenum). Here, it acts as a detergent, breaking down dietary fat globules into an emulsion of tiny droplets that are easier to absorb. If you don't have a gallbladder, bile trickles down into the duodenum continuously which sometimes causes problems such as bloating or loose bowels from poor digestion of dietary fats.

Every day, your liver produces between 750ml and 1500ml of bile fluid which contains water, bile pigments (bilirubin and biliverdin), bile acid salts (80% of which are sodium glycholate and sodium taurocholate derived from cholic acid), cholesterol and phospholipids such as lecithin (phosphatidylcholine).

> **Did you know?** Bile pigments are yellow (bilirubin) or green (biliverdin). Bacteria in your large bowel convert these to the more familiar brown colour found in faeces. If bile outflow from the liver is blocked, bilirubin will build up in your blood to cause jaundice and your faeces will develop a pale, putty colour.

The presence of gallstones affects how well your gallbladder contracts. Those classed as 'bad contractors' have severely impaired or even absent gallbladder emptying. Even 'good contractors' may retain more bile after a meal, or when fasting, compared with

123

normal, however. This retention of bile further adds to the growth of existing stones and the formation of new ones. It also increases the risk of Candida colonising the gallbladder.

One of the best ways to increase bile production in order to suppress Candida growth in the biliary tract and small intestines, is to take globe artichoke (*Cynara scolymus*) leaf supplements.

Curcumin also boosts liver function, stimulates secretion of bile and is widely used to treat gallbladder/biliary dysfunction. It induces contraction of the gall-bladder and can reduce biliary pain – see under the Repair section, later.

Re-inoculate

The Re-inoculate phase of the 5Rs approach involves replenishing levels of friendly digestive bacteria.

Your large intestines contain around 11 trillion bacteria, weighing a total of 1.5 kg. Ideally, at least 70 per cent of these should be 'friendly' acid-producing probiotic bacteria and only 30 per cent other gas-forming bowel bacteria such as E. coli. In practice, however, the balance is usually the other way round.

Probiotic bacteria play an important role in maintaining a healthy intestinal balance and keeping Candida yeasts at bay. They produce lactic and acetic acids which discourage the growth of potentially harmful bacteria, secrete natural antibiotics (bacteriocins) and stimulate production of antiviral interferons. They also compete with harmful bacteria and yeasts for available nutrients, and for attachment sites on intestinal cell walls so that other microorganisms such as Candida are less likely to take hold. Another benefit is that probiotic bacteria produce short-chain fatty acids (eg butyrate) which, act as a major energy source for intestinal lining cells. These fatty acids are also absorbed from the colon and transported to the liver where they have a positive effect on bile production and cholesterol metabolism.

Re-inoculating your bowel with 'friendly' digestive bacteria is an important step in overcoming Candida.

The term *probiotic* literally means 'for life' and probiotics are defined by the World Health Organisation as 'live micro-organisms which, when administered in adequate amounts, confer a health benefit on the host'. The most commonly used probiotic organisms are certain strains of Lactobacillus (eg *L. acidophilus*, *L. reuteri*, *L. casei*, *L. rhamnosus*, *L. plantarum 299v*) and Bifidobacter (eg *B. bifidum*, *B. infantis*, *B. lactis*, *B. longum*, *B. breve*). Even a yeast, *Saccharomyces boulardii*, is accepted as having probiotic properties. Because these probiotics are acid tolerant, a significant number survive passage through the stomach to reach and colonise the large intestines.

Probiotic lactic-acid producing bacteria that are naturally found in the gut are believed to inhibit the growth of Candida yeasts, to improve IBS-like intestinal symptoms and to reduce the chance of yeasts being transferred to the genital tract to cause vaginal thrush. Studies show, for example, that taking both probiotics and the antifungal drug, fluconazole, can significantly improve treatment response with less discharge and lower presence of vaginal yeasts.

Probiotic bacteria are found in fermented foods such as live 'Bio' yogurts, cottage cheese, miso, kefir and tempeh while numerous probiotic supplements are available.

The term *prebiotics* refers to non-digestible food ingredients that selectively feed the growth of prebiotic bacteria in the colon. These cannot be used as a food source by other, less beneficial bacteria, including *E. coli*. Prebiotics include substances known as fructo-oligosaccharides (FOS) and inulin. These prebiotic fibres are found in foods such as oats, barley, wheat, garlic, onions, leeks, bananas, honey, tomatoes, Jerusalem artichokes, globe artichokes, asparagus, shiitake mushrooms, aubergine, rocket, chicory and edamame soy beans.

Probiotics and prebiotics are now increasingly used together, in a practice known as *synbiotics* to reinoculate the bowel with friendly digestive bacteria and supress gas-forming bacteria and yeasts. Taking probiotic supplements to replenish the normal balance of bacteria in the bowel has been shown to:
• restore normal intestinal permeability
• overcome leaky gut syndrome
• improve liver function

- reduce inflammatory immune reactions associated with atopic conditions such as eczema, asthma and allergic rhinitis
- reduce recurrent attacks of vaginal thrush.

Dose: Select a supplement supplying a known quantity of probiotic bacteria such as 5 billion or 20 billion colony forming units (CFU) per dose. Enteric coated supplements, which improve survival of probiotic bacteria as they pass through the stomach, can contain less (eg 10 million CFU) and still provide beneficial effects.

Check the shelf life - supplements close to their expiry date contain fewer live probiotic bacteria than those with a longer shelf life. Also check whether it needs refrigeration. Freeze-dried bacteria, which are held in suspended animation, do not need to be kept chilled.

Repair

The Repair phase of the 5Rs approach involves supplements that promote the healing of a damaged or inflamed intestinal lining. These include vitamin D, omega-3 fatty acids, the amino acid L-glutamine, and curcumin extracted from turmeric spice. Other micronutrients important for the integrity of the bowel lining include vitamins A, C, B5 and E, plus antioxidant carotenoids and zinc.

Repair with additional vitamin D

Lack of vitamin D is common, especially during winter in northern climes, as you only make vitamin D from the action of sunlight on your skin when the UV index is greater than 3. Vitamin D deficiency compromises the integrity of the gut lining, contributing to 'leaky gut syndrome' and may increase the risk of developing inflammatory bowel disease. Lack of vitamin D is also linked with reduced immunity and an increased change of developing bacterial vaginosis – an imbalance of vaginal bacteria that promotes Candida overgrowth. The usual dose is 25mcg to 100mcg daily (see Chapter 3).

Repair with omega-3 fatty acids

Fish oils are a rich source of two long-chain, omega-3 polyunsaturated fatty acids: eicosapentaenoic acid (EPA) and docosahexaenoic acid (DHA). These are converted in the body into substances (series 3 prostaglandins and series 5 leukotrienes) that reduce inflammation. This helps to balance the action of omega-6 fatty acids (mostly derived from vegetables oils such as safflower, corn and sunflower oils) which are converted into substances that promote inflammation. Omega-3s therefore offer some benefit against long-term inflammatory conditions including intestinal inflammation.

Omega-3 fish oils are extracted from the flesh of oily fish such as salmon, herrings, sardines, pilchards and mackerel. These beneficial oils are derived from the micro-algae on which the fish feed. Long-chain omega-3 supplements are therefore available from algae extracts, as well as from fish oils. Vegetarians and vegans should select algae-derived omega-3s as these are in the beneficial long-chain form, not flax seed supplements which supply short-chain omega-3s (only 5% of these are converted on to the beneficial long-chain omega-3s in the body).

To avoid essential fatty acid deficiency, you need the equivalent of 450mg long-chain omega 3 fish oils (DHA and EPA) per day (at least 3g per week). However, the average adult only eats 1/3rd of a portion of oily fish, supplying a meagre 1g fish oils per week, and 70% of adults eat no oily fish at all.

As diet should always come first, concentrate on eating at least two portions of oily fish per week. The typical amount of long-chain omega-3s these supply is shown in the following table.

Fish	Portion (grams)	Long-chain omega-3s per portion (grams)
Kippers	150g	3.89g
Salmon	150g	3.25g
Mackerel	150g	2.89g
Pilchards in tomato sauce	110g	2.86g
Herring	150g	1.97g
Tuna (fresh)	150g	1.95g
Trout	150g	1.73g
Sardines in tomato sauce	100g	1.67g

Salmon (canned in brine)	100g	1.55g
Plaice	150g	0.45g
Cod	150g	0.38g
Haddock	150g	0.24g
Tuna (in oil, drained)	45g	0.17g
Tuna (in brine, drained)	45g	0.08g

If selecting a fish oil supplements, some evidence suggests that Krill oil is the best form as it has optimum levels of EPA and DHA, and the oils are present in a phospholipid form that aids fat digestion, liver health, bile flow and cell membrane function.

At the same time as increasing your intake of long-chain omega-3s, aim to cut back on the omega-6 fats that promote inflammation by consuming less:

- vegetable oils (except olive, flaxseed, walnut, almond, macadamia, avocado, hempseed and rapeseed oils which contain omega-3s and/or monounsaturated fats)
- meat
- margarines
- convenience and fast-foods
- manufactured goods such as biscuits, cakes, sweets and pastries.

Dose: Omega-3 fish oils: 1g to 4g a day. Typically a 1g capsule of high-strength fish oil contains around 500mg of the important long-chain omega-3 fatty acids, EPA and DHA (check label claims).

Krill oil: 300 mg to 3 g daily.

Cod liver oil: 1g - 1.5g per day. If choosing to take cod liver oil, those described as high or extra high strength provide the highest amount of omega-3 fatty acids. If taking a multivitamin as well, check the total amounts of vitamin A and D you are taking do not exceed recommended doses. Vitamin A is best limited to less than 5,000 IU (1,500 mcg) per day although intakes of up to 10,000 IU (3,000 mcg) are considered safe. Vitamin D intakes should not normally excess 100mcg (4000 IU) per day (except under medical advice).

> *NB Cod liver oil products should not be taken during pregnancy as they contain vitamin A, an excess of which is harmful to a developing baby.*

Because of their blood thinning properties, people with clotting disorders or who are taking blood-thinning medication such as warfarin should only take an omega-3 fish oil supplement under supervision by a doctor. However, no significant increase in blood clotting time is expected at total daily intakes of EPA and DHA of 3g per day, or less.

Repair with l-glutamine

L-glutamine is an amino acid synthesised in the body which becomes in short supply – and therefore essential from the diet - during times of stress, and when recovering from injury, infection or surgery.

> *Did you know?* *Food sources of l-glutamine include lean proteins such as fish, chicken, lamb and fresh meat stocks and broths. Once heated above 40 degrees, however, l-glutamine becomes inactive. Its precursor, glutamic acid, from which it is made in the body is present in grains, grapes, nuts and chocolate.*

L-glutamine has several important roles in metabolism - including the production of brain neurotransmitters, helping to overcome mental fatigue, anxiety and lift mood. L-glutamine is also vital for the production of genetic material in rapidly dividing cells, especially immune cells and those lining the gut. It is used as the preferred fuel for enterocytes – the cells lining the gut which act as a barrier against infection. L-glutamine supplements have been shown to:

• Increase the height of villi, the finger-like projections in the small intestine through which nutrients are absorbed into the circulation

• Stimulate the growth and proliferation of cells lining the gut (mucosal layer)

• Maintain the integrity of the mucosal barrier

• Prevent intestinal leakiness and the movement of gut bacteria into the tissues (bacterial translocation).

If l-glutamine is in short supply, the intestinal lining becomes increasingly permeable and when l-glutamine was first discovered it was initially referred to as 'intestinal permeability factor'. L-glutamine supplements are used to reduce permeability of the gut in people with inflammatory bowel conditions such as ulcerative colitis or Crohn's disease. Although studies have shown conflicting results, one study in which ulcerative colitis patients were given 30 g of glutamine daily, for four weeks, produced significant clinical and endoscopic improvements, which worsened when the supplements were stopped.

Dose: 5g to 30g per day

Repair with Aloe vera

Aloe vera leaves provide a gel that contains vitamins, minerals, antioxidants, amino acids, anthraquinones, saponins and natural plant steroids with a soothing, anti-inflammatory action. It contains a fibroblast growth factor that hastens wound healing, antiseptics with antibacterial, anti-viral and anti-fungal properties, plus soothing analgesics (eg salicylic acid).

Aloe vera juice appears to boost immunity, and is used for a variety of intestinal problems, including indigestion, constipation, irritable bowel syndrome (IBS) and inflammatory bowel conditions such as ulcerative colitis and Crohn's disease.

Did you know? Some *Aloe vera* products contain a bitter aloe *'latex'* extracted from the inner yellow leaves of the plant. This can cause a brisk, laxative response due to the presence of anthraquinones (aloin, emodin). These stimulate bowel contraction and usually work within 8–12 hours. If this laxative response is not required, select products that are certified aloin/emodin free (eg stamped with an IASC-certified seal from the International Aloe Science Council).

Dose: If taking aloe latex for its laxative effect, start with a small dose of gel (e.g. 1 teaspoon) and work up to around 1–2 tablespoons per day to find which dose suits you best.

Aloe vera juice is taken more liberally (e.g. 50–100 ml, three times daily). When selecting a product, aim for one made from 100 per cent pure *Aloe vera*. Its strength needs to be at least 40 per cent by volume to be effective and should ideally approach 95–100 per cent. You may find it more palatable to choose a product containing a little natural fruit juice (e.g. grape, apple) to improve the flavour.

Some women using *Aloe vera* may notice increased menstrual flow, but no serious side effects have been reported at standard doses.

Do not take *Aloe vera* during pregnancy (despite the fact that it is often promoted by manufacturer) as it can stimulate uterine contractions which could result in miscarriage. *Aloe vera* aloin also enters breast milk and can trigger stomach cramps and diarrhoea in infants.

Repair with curcumin

Curcumin is the powerful, anti-inflammatory that gives turmeric spice its rich yellow colour. Curcumin stimulates secretion of bile and boosts liver regeneration and function by increasing levels of two liver enzymes: glutathione-s-transferase and glucuronyl transferase.

In 207 people with symptoms compatible with irritable bowel syndrome (IBS) which are similar to those associated with Candida, symptoms halved in those taking 1g turmeric daily for 8 weeks, and improved by 60% in those taking 2g daily. Placebo controlled trials are needed to confirm its effectiveness, however.

In 89 people with ulcerative colitis, taking 1g curcumin twice a day for 6 months during a period of remission (in addition to their usual medication) significantly reduced the chance of a relapse of bowel inflammation (4.6% relapse rate in those taking curcumin versus 20.5% of those taking inactive placebo). Taking curcumin also improved the findings on endoscopy, suggesting that it is an effective treatment for bowel inflammation

Recent research suggests that curcumin works by inserting itself into intestinal cell membranes to stabilise them and improve their resistance to infection and inflammation. See Chapter 3.

Rebalance

The Re-balancing phase of the 5Rs approach involves adopting a healthier diet and lifestyle going forwards. In general, this means following a so-called alkaline diet with plenty of fruit and vegetables, lean protein and fibre with minimal processed and sugary foods, additives and preservatives.

Rebalance with an alkaline diet

There is a lot of confusion around the concept of 'acid' and 'alkaline' foods. These terms refer to the effects eating these foods have on your urine, and are not based on whether or not the food itself is acidic. All foods trigger production of hydrochloric acid in the stomach (assuming you can make sufficient amounts) and all foods trigger the production of strongly alkaline secretions from the pancreas and small intestines, so food has little effect on the pH of your digestive tract overall. Similarly, foods have little effect on the acidity of your blood, which is normally tightly regulated within a narrow pH range that is slightly alkaline (pH 7.35 - 7.45). In fact, if your blood pH falls more than 0.5 units either side of 7.4 you will become seriously ill as your cells and metabolic enzymes need a constant, low level of alkalinity to work properly.

When foods are described as having an 'acid' or 'alkaline' effect, this relates to the effect they have on the pH of your urine after they are fully processed in your body. When food is broken down, its various building blocks – amino acids, carbohydrates, fatty acids – are metabolised to either generate or consume acid units called protons. Protons are the positively charged hydrogen ions (H+) whose concentration determines the pH of a fluid.

If the metabolism of a particular food results in the production of excess protons it is classified as an 'acid' food.

If the metabolism of a particular food uses up more protons than it produces, it is classified as an 'alkaline' food.

Although some foods such as oranges, lemons, limes and tomatoes taste acidic, the way their building blocks are metabolised uses up acid so they are classified as 'alkaline' foods. In fact, fruit is your main dietary source of alkali as they contain the sodium and potassium salts of weak organic acids. During metabolism, these weak acids are lost when you produce carbon dioxide – an acidic gas which you breathe out via your lungs to eliminate acidity. This leaves behind sodium and potassium bicarbonate which are alkaline, so most fruit and vegetables are alkaline-forming foods.

Similarly, although raw meat is slightly alkaline (because it contains blood with a pH of 7.4) the metabolism of amino acids produces an excess of acidity. Most of this is lost from the body in the form of acidic carbon dioxide gas, but some of the excess acid is voided in your urine. Meat is therefore classed as an 'acid-forming' food.

Naturopaths suggest eating a diet that consists of 70% - 80% alkaline-forming foods and only 20% - 30% acid-forming foods, so you can still have some foods like pasta and white rice, but in moderation.

The most important alkaline-forming foods, which you can generally consume freely (unless you are intolerant to them) include:

Mildly Alkaline:	Low sugar fruits, berries, peppers, limes, lemons, grapefruit
Strongly Alkaline:	Green leafy vegetables, kale, broccoli, spinach, avocado, tomato

The most important acid forming foods to consume in moderation are:

Mildly acidic:	Grains (barley, oats, quinoa, rice, wheat, bread), Pulses (eg black beans, chickpeas, kidney beans, lentils), Nuts (pecans, cashews, peanuts, pistachios, walnuts), Some fruits (eg blueberries, cranberries, plums, prunes, fruit juices), Dairy products (cream, cheese, milk, ice-cream, yogurt)
Strongly acidic:	Animal proteins (eggs, poultry, meats, seafood), Beer, Coffee, Fruit juice (sweetened), Tea

Alkaline cookbooks are available to provide nutritious, tasty recipes. One I particularly like is 'Honestly Healthy For Life' by gourmet vegetarian chef Natasha Corrett and nutritional therapist Vicki Edgson. This includes over 100 alkaline recipes, including

Pumpkin and Orange Risotto, Melt-in-the-mouth Doughnuts and even Sticky Toffee Pudding – the healthy way – for those not tightly restricting their sugar intake.

Acid-forming foods are important dietary sources of protein, vitamins, minerals, antioxidants and other nutrients. If you plan to adopt this approach long-term, seek advice from of a qualified medical nutritionist who will tell you how to how best to replace these nutrients in your diet. For example, if you plan to follow a mainly vegetarian or vegan diet, you need to support your intake of vitamins B12 and D, iron, and zinc.

Rebalance with a traditional anti-Candida diet

Although some people view the anti-Candida diet with suspicion, it has undoubtedly helped many people with symptoms thought to be due to candidiasis. There is little to lose by following an anti-Candida regime for a few weeks to see if it helps you.

A basic anti-Candida diet involves avoiding excess sugars and products containing brewers' or bakers' yeast as these can cross-react to cause problems for those with yeast intolerance or Candida hypersensitivity syndrome. Instructions usually suggest avoiding:

• White or brown sugar and food or drinks containing these (eg honey, jam, desserts, treacle, syrups, cakes, biscuits, sauces, ice-cream, soft drinks, dried fruits, chocolates, malt).

- Refined (processed) carbohydrates (eg white flour, white rice) and products made from them (eg biscuits, cakes, buns, white bread).
- Products containing yeasts or moulds such as yeast extracts, cheese, bread made with yeast, alcoholic drinks, vinegar and pickled foods, smoked foods, soy sauce, tofu, grapes and grape juice, unpeeled fruits, dried fruits, frozen or concentrated fruit juices, old potentially mouldy foods and vegetables, mushrooms, B vitamin supplements that are not labelled 'yeast-free'.
- Some sugar substitutes such as sorbitol, mannitol, xylitol, aspartame and saccharin which are metabolised like alcohol to produce substances that may stimulate Candida growth.
- Alcohol, tea, coffee, cocoa products, malted night-time drinks, fizzy drinks, fruit squashes.

It may take a few days for a change in diet to affect your symptoms. If your problems are not significantly improved within two to three weeks of following a restrictive anti-Candida diet, it is important to return to eating a wider range of foods to guard against any nutrient deficiencies. If you are able to identify a small number of foods that undoubtedly provoke your symptoms however, these can usually be avoided without affecting your overall nutrition.

Rebalance by avoiding stress

Even mild stress reduces the integrity of your intestinal lining and suppresses secretion of digestive enzymes and IgA antibodies which are vital for immune protection in the gut. This is because the stress-related 'fight or flight' response slows digestion, shunts blood away from the gut towards muscles and raises blood glucose levels as part of your primitive survival response. The shutting down of digestion allows partially digested food to start putrefying in the bowel – a perfect substrate for Candida yeasts to feed on. Raised glucose levels in the tissues along with suppressed immune responses, may also support Candida growth.

Keep a stress diary to work out what stresses you most in life. Keep your diary close to hand so you can jot things down after each stressful event. Record how you feel at the time and when you later recognise a negative responses that was triggered by the event, note this down, too. Having identified a stressor, think about possible solutions to help you cope more successfully if the stressful event recurs. Sometimes, it's as easy as not shopping after work when the supermarket is busy – plan to go at a quieter time, or have groceries delivered to home or work. If commuting to work during rush hour stresses you, can you negotiate flexihours, or working at least some of the week from home? Avoidance is not always appropriate however - you can't avoid a colleague who causes you stress at work. These situations are best dealt with by changing how you respond to them. Going out of your way to genuinely be nice or helpful to someone, even if you don't like them, often pays unexpected dividends.

If stress results from events that happen around you, what can you do to change them? For example, if you view a change imposed on you as a threat (eg redundancy) how can you turn this into an

141

opportunity (eg retrain to solidify another skill into career path you've always fancied but never had time to explore).

Some causes of stress are internal, and may result from lifestyle choices (eg working or playing too hard leading to physical tiredness, mental exhaustion), lack of fitness, hormone changes (eg menstruation, menopause), disrupted bio-rhythms (eg working shifts) or negative self-image and thoughts. If you think you aren't good enough, or that you won't be able to cope, these become self-fulfilling prophecies. If you believe you ARE good enough, and are determined to cope then you will keep trying until you succeed.

Here are some relatively simple things you can do to reduce stress:

Consider your work-life balance and plan to spend more time with those you love, doing things you love.

Schedule regular relaxation breaks into your day: a powernap if you are tired, a meditation to clear your mind, a walk around the park if you are stuck behind a desk all day.

Stop clock-watching – try not wearing a watch, and don't stress over less important deadlines. In most cases, you can renegotiate and extend a deadline with little risk of disaster.

Draw up a plan to delegate or share more responsibilities at home and/or work.

Don't look for excuses to be disappointed in yourself or others –
instead, look for excuses to say 'well done' or 'thank you'. Big up
your successes rather than minimising them.

Talk about your emotions rather than bottling them up. Explain to
family, friends and work colleagues how you feel. It is important to
be clear in what you are saying, so think this through beforehand.

Don't judge yourself too harshly. Accept you are doing your best.
Write down 10 things you like about yourself.

Make molehills out of mountains, rather than the other way round
by avoiding words that exaggerate events. Instead of saying
'terrible' say 'inconvenient', instead of 'dreadful' say 'annoying',
for 'awful' try 'unfortunate' and in place of 'I have to...' use 'I
would like to'. Replace 'I must...' with 'I intend to...'

> **Did you know?** An ancient Chinese technique is great for relieving
> stress. Imagine something that makes you smile, and smile internally
> so it is only felt by you. It doesn't have to be visible. Let the smile
> shine out of your eyes and travel inwards to spread all over your
> body before concentrating the feeling just below your navel. As the
> smile radiates within, it generates a lovely feeling of relaxation and
> peace.

Practise mindfulness meditation in which you focus on the present
moment. Paying close attention to everyday activities such as
preparing food or walking and concentrating on the sensations,
textures, colours, smells and sounds involved, helps to prevent your
mind spinning off and dwelling on potentially negative and stressful
thoughts.

143

Tune into your inner 'sound of silence' which resembles a high-pitched, constant tone at the periphery of your consciousness. Once you are aware of it, and know how to find it, you can access it at any time (even in noisy surroundings) to help you relax when feeling stressed.

Explore what relaxation classes are available in your area, such as yoga and meditation.

Consider your overall health. Make an appointment with your doctor to have your blood pressure, glucose, cholesterol and thyroid hormone levels checked. Take a urine sample with you for glucose screening - especially if you are experiencing recurrent thrush and haven't had a diabetes screen within the last six months.

CHAPTER 3

Nutritional Supplements

A number of supplements are used to help overcome recurrent Candida. These work in different ways and may:
- Boost your natural immunity
- Overcome the adverse effects of stress that suppresses immunity
- Suppress yeast growth without killing them (fungistatic) buying time for your immune system to get on top of the infection
- Kill yeasts directly (fungicidal).

If you have a medical condition or are taking any prescribed drugs, always check with a doctor or pharmacist before taking a supplement.

> *Do not take any supplements during pregnant or breast-feeding unless a doctor advises that the benefits are likely to outweigh the risks.*

Vitamin C

Vitamin C (ascorbic acid) is a water-soluble vitamin which cannot be stored in the body. As it is needed for at least 300 metabolic reactions, including those involved in immunity and healing, a regular dietary intake is essential. Food sources include most fruit and vegetables especially citrus, berries, blackcurrants, capsicum peppers, kiwi fruit and green leafy vegetables.

> **Did you know?** *Vitamin C increases the absorption of dietary iron. When taking iron supplements, wash them down with a glass of fresh orange juice.*

Lack of vitamin C reduces immunity and increases your susceptibility to recurrent Candida and other infections. During times of stress, your vitamin C needs increase significantly as part of your fight-or flight reaction, which at least doubles your normal requirements. Vitamin C also acts as an antioxidant in all body tissues, helping to reduce inflammation. It is rapidly used up to neutralise the oxidative stress associated with vaginal thrush and loss of its antioxidant protection may increase the level of inflammation (soreness, redness and swelling) present.

Research findings

A study involving 257 women with vaginitis (inflammation of the vagina) due to Candida, bacterial vaginosis (a common bacterial imbalance) or trichomoniasis (a protozoal infection) confirmed that vitamin C levels decrease before treatment then increase again after successful treatment.

New research, published in 2014, shows that vitamin C inhibits the switching of *Candida albicans* from the smooth, harmless cell form to the active form that produces invasive threads. This is supported by a study that investigated nutritional deficiencies in elderly hospitalised patients. Those with oral candidiasis were significantly more likely to have a low vitamin C level than a similar group without oral Candida. The researchers concluded that vitamin C deficiency is as important a risk factor for oral Candida as taking antibiotics, poor oral hygiene and wearing dentures.

Dose

Experts in different countries suggest vitamin C intakes that vary from 40mg to 120 mg/day to meet the requirements of a healthy population. The upper safe level for long-term use from supplements is suggested as 1000mg (1g).

The absorption and metabolism of vitamin C depends on the amount consumed. At intakes of up to 200 mg/day as a single dose, absorption of vitamin C is almost complete through an active transport process. At single doses of over 500 mg, it is also absorbed through a process of diffusion, but efficiency of absorption declines as doses increase, so that only half of a 1.5g dose is absorbed (ie 750mg).

For people with active thrush, I normally suggest a minimum intake of 1g per day, and up to 1g three times daily, for short-term use, if you can tolerate it without diarrhoea or indigestion. The form

147

known as ester-C is 'body-ready', non-acidic and most easily tolerated.

If you are taking high doses of vitamin C and need to have a urine test, inform your doctor as taking supplements can affect laboratory results. Some urine test kits used by diabetics are affected by high dose vitamin C, for example – use a kit that is not affected.

People with iron-storage disease (haemochromatosis) should only take vitamin C supplements under medical advice.

Recurrent kidney stone formers, and those with kidney failure who may have a defect in ascorbic acid or oxalate metabolism, should restrict daily vitamin C intakes to approximately 100 mg daily.

Cut back on a high dose of vitamin C slowly, over the course of a week or two, once the Candida episode is resolved, rather than stopping suddenly. This avoids a so-called 'rebound scurvy' effect in which enzymes activated by high levels of vitamin C are suddenly deprived of the extra vitamin C they need to work properly. This can produce temporary symptoms of vitamin C deficiency.

Vitamin D

Vitamin D is a fat-soluble vitamin that occurs in five different forms, the most important of which are vitamin D2 (ergocalciferol derived from plants) and vitamin D3 (cholecalciferol derived from animals). Vitamin D3 is the most important for immune health and whenever I mention vitamin D, assume I mean vitamin D3. Food sources include oily fish, fish liver oils, animal liver, fortified margarine, eggs, butter and fortified milk, as shown in the following table:

Food	Vitamin D content
Herring (3oz)	1400 IU
Sardines (3.5oz)	500 IU
Mackerel (3.5oz)	350 IU
Salmon (3.5oz)	350 IU
Tuna (3oz)	200 IU
Full fat milk (250ml)	100 IU
Whole egg	20 IU

You make some vitamin D in your skin from a reaction involving ultraviolet light when the UV index is greater than 3. There is a wide seasonal and regional variation in the amount of vitamin D produced by people in different countries. Those living at a latitude of 520N (which passes through the centre of the UK and Canada) receive too little UVB radiation to make vitamin D between the months of October and April. Those living at a latitude 420N (which forms the northern limit of Spain and part of the border between Canada and North America) are unable to synthesis vitamin D between November to February. Low vitamin D status is therefore widespread at northern latitudes, and, with the exception

149

of Norway (where intakes of vitamin-D rich fish are high) most Europeans have low vitamin D levels during winter.

Vitamin D levels are also low in those who habitually wear clothes that cover most of their skin, or who stay indoors most of the time.

To balance adequate production of vitamin D against skin cancer risk from excess UV exposure, usual advice is to obtain 10 to 15 minutes sunlight on face, arms, hands or back, two or three times a week, without sunscreen. Fifteen minutes exposure to strong sunlight can produce as much as 10,000 IU vitamin D in your skin, but some people do not make or handle vitamin D efficiently. Longer exposures do not provide additional benefit, as skin vitamin D is rapidly degraded by excess UV radiation.

> ***Did you know?*** *Used properly, a sunscreen with a sun protection factor of 8 reduces your vitamin D production by 95%, while SPF15 reduces vitamin D production by 99%. Most people do not apply enough sunscreen, however, and the development of a tan suggests that enough UVB radiation strikes the skin to stimulate production of both melanin (a natural sunscreen produced in response to UV damage) and some vitamin D regardless of sunscreen use.*

Vitamin D protects against Candida and other infections by helping to maintain the integrity of your intestinal lining and protecting against infection. Vitamin D receptors are present in the nucleus of most immune cells, including the T lymphocytes, neutrophils and macrophages, where it switches on genes needed to fight invaders. A good vitamin D intakes ensure rapid immune responses, including antibody production.

150

Research findings

White blood cells (neutrophils) from people with an hereditary defect in vitamin D production are up to 40% less able to kill Candida yeasts than those from people with normal vitamin D levels. Little else was known about the effects of vitamin D on immune responses to Candida until 2011, however, when a small study involving 14 healthy volunteers showed that taking vitamin D3 supplements significantly improved the ability of immune cells to recognise *Candida albicans* infection, and reduced the resulting inflammatory response.

Vitamin D reduces the risk of a bacterial imbalance that promotes Candida overgrowth. Bacterial vaginosis (BV) is associated with low or absent numbers of beneficial 'probiotic' bacteria in the vagina. This allows the overgrowth of anaerobic bacteria (which thrive in low oxygen environments) and Candida yeasts. Some studies suggest that as many as one in four women have bacterial vaginosis at any one time. BV often arises spontaneously around the time of menstruation, then resolves mid-cycle although recurrences are common. The exact cause is unknown, and it is not classed as a sexually transmissible disease although it is more common in sexually active women. The chemicals produced by anaerobic bacteria make the normally acid vaginal secretions more alkaline, and release an ammonia-like smell that has been likened to rotting fish. The fishy odour is worse after unprotected sex when the discharge is mixed with alkaline semen, and also after urination if it mixes with alkaline urine.

The chemicals produced in BV can cause mild irritation and increased watery discharge. Around fifty percent of women with BV do not get appreciable symptoms, however. Male partners may develop irritation after sex if they have not used a condom, but treating male contacts does not seem to reduce the risk of recurrences in their female partners.

If you suspect you may have BV, this can be diagnosed and treated at a sexual health (genito-urinary) clinic. Treatment involves antibiotics such as metronidazole tablets/gel or clindamycin cream or using an acid-based gel (from pharmacies). To help prevent recurrences of BV, it may help to take a probiotic supplement, to use probiotic pessaries and/or to take vitamin D supplements.

Dose

As so many factors influence your vitamin D requirement, it is a good idea to have a blood test to assess your individual level. This will show whether or not you need to take a supplement.

Many people who are vitamin D deficient do not significantly boost their blood level by taking a 10mcg (400IU) supplement. Some experts suggest that, in the absences of exposure to sunlight, a minimum daily intake of 20mcg (800 IU) vitamin D is needed to maintain a healthy blood level during winter months. Others argue that an intake of 40 mcg per day (1600 IU) is needed - irrespective of sun exposure.

If you have recurrent Candida, it seems sensible to take at least 40mcg per day (1600 IU). The accepted upper safe level for long-term use from supplements was recently increased to 100 mcg vitamin D per day (4000 IU) so you could take up to this level if you wish, for eight weeks, and then have your level rechecked.

Look for supplements supplying vitamin D3 (cholecalciferol) as this is 20% to 40% more effective in maintaining blood vitamin D levels than the vitamin D2 (ergocalciferol or plant) form.

Did you know? *200 IU vitamin D is equivalent to 5 mcg.*

Toxic effects can occur at intakes exceeding 500 mcg vitamin D per day, including headache, loss of appetite, nausea, vomiting, diarrhoea or constipation, palpitations and fatigue.

Biotin

Biotin is a water-soluble member of the vitamin B group. It is an essential co-factor for four enzymes involved in the metabolism of glucose and the synthesis of stress hormones, and plays a role in maintaining the strength and integrity of skin, hair and nails.

Biotin is widespread in the diet and good sources include meat, liver, oily fish, whole grains, rice, nuts, cauliflower, egg yolk and yeast extracts. It is also produced by probiotic bacteria in the bowel, from which it can be absorbed. Dietary deficiency of biotin is therefore unusual, except in those following a very low-calorie weight loss diet and in those eating large amounts of raw egg white over a long period (eg body builders) - raw egg white contains a protein, avidin, which binds to biotin in the gut and prevents its absorption. Cooked egg white does not have this effect.

> *Did you know?* Those on long-term antibiotic treatment are at higher risk of biotin deficiency due to loss of the normal probiotic bowel bacteria that make it. Taking a probiotic supplement when on antibiotics will help to overcome this.

Research findings

When biotin is lacking, the strength of hair, nails and skin is affected, and a characteristic red, scaly rash develops around body orifices. *Candida albicans* can often be cultured from these skin lesions. An estimated one in 123 people has an inherited inborn error of biotin metabolism due to impaired intestinal absorption. This reduces the activity and effectiveness of T-cell and B-cells needed to fight yeast infections and allows yeasts to penetrate weakened skin and nails. If you have recurrent Candida, and have weak, soft nails that split easily, you may benefit from a biotin supplement.

Dose

The average need for biotin is between 50mcg and 150mcg per day. Supplements with doses as high as 5,000mcg and 10,000 mcg are available for short-term use under the advice of a nutritional therapist. However, the upper safe level for long-term use from supplements is suggested as 900 mcg.

Two out of three people respond to even low dose biotin supplements with significantly improved nail growth, suggesting that some degree of deficiency is common. It's certainly worth trying if you have recurrent candidiasis.

Iron

Iron is an essential mineral best known for its role in carrying oxygen within the red blood pigment, haemoglobin. Dietary iron comes in two main forms: protein-bound haem iron from animal sources such as fish, shellfish, red meats and egg yolk, and mineral (inorganic) iron from plant sources such as wholemeal bread, green vegetables, dried fruit and enriched cereals. Haem iron is 'body ready' and absorbed via a specific haem receptor three times more efficiently than non-haem iron. However, most dietary iron is obtained in inorganic form, 48% from cereal products, 16% from vegetables. However, over boiling vegetables decreases their iron availability by up to 20 per cent.

Did you know? Inorganic iron exists in two oxidation states as ferrous ($Fe2+$) and ferric ($Fe3+$) ions which have separate uptake mechanisms. Ferric iron – the form in which most plant-derived iron is obtained - is less well absorbed due to low solubility at higher pH. Vitamin C increases iron absorption by converting ferric iron to ferrous iron.

Dietary iron deficiency is common and, worldwide, is the most common nutritional disease. Low iron intakes lead to the production of red blood cells that are smaller and paler than normal due to lack of haemoglobin. A low-grade iron deficiency impairs immunity even if frank iron-deficiency anaemia (IDA) is not present. Those most at risk include:

- Infants who are exclusively breast-fed (formulas/follow-on milks are fortified)
- Toddlers - studies suggest 28% have low iron stores, and 12% to 30% have IDA
- Adolescents – 64% have low iron stores and 20% have IDA
- Menstruating women - 32% have low iron stores, 11% have no stores and 36% have IDA
- Pregnant women
- Non-meat eaters
- The elderly – up to 10% living at home have IDA and the prevalence is higher in institutions.

White blood cells use an array of powerful, iron-containing chemicals to destroy invading micro-organisms (bacteria, yeasts, viruses). Candida yeasts need iron themselves to grow properly and your white blood cells (neutrophils) release an iron-binding protein, called lactoferrin, to clears iron from your tissues as a first-line defence against Candida. However, *Candida albicans*.has evolved at least three systems to help them thrive when iron levels are low, however, one of which involves suppressing their production of genes that code for iron-dependent proteins. These mechanisms ensure it can still overgrow when your own iron levels are depleted, and recurrent thrush is often one of the first signs of iron deficiency seen in general practice.

Research findings

A 2013 study investigated the possible effects of iron deficiency on recurrent vulvovaginal candidiasis. Ninety-two women were divided into four groups based on whether or not they had recurrent Candida and/or iron-deficiency anaemia. Their immune function was assessed using the activity of two types of immune T-helper cells, Th1 and Th2. Previous studies suggested that a response predominantly involving Th1 boosts resistance against recurrent vulvovaginal candidiasis, while a response mainly involving Th2 cells exacerbates the degree of inflammation and symptoms. The research confirmed that the presence of iron-deficiency anaemia changes the balance towards a Th2 response which could contribute to reduced immunity and worsening inflammation in recurrent candidiasis.

The only way to detect iron deficiency when iron deficiency anaemia itself is not present is to measure your circulating levels of the iron binding protein, ferritin. If you haven't had this done, ask your doctor to check this for you.

Dose

The EU RDA for iron is 14 mg for adults. The upper safe level for long-term use from supplements is only slightly higher, at 17mg per day as it is such as potentially toxic metal. Don't take higher amounts unless your doctor prescribes them for proven iron-deficiency anaemia. Excess iron can cause constipation or indigestion and excess is toxic (especially for children – keep supplements out of their reach – eating just a few has been fatal for toddlers.)

As taking iron supplements decreases absorption of zinc and other essential minerals (such as manganese, chromium and selenium) it's usually advisable to take iron as part of an A to Z multivitamin and mineral supplement (unless prescribed individually by a doctor).

Supplements containing iron in the ferrous (not the ferric) form are preferable. Of these, ferrous fumarate and ferrous gluconate are usually better tolerated than ferrous sulphate.

Iron-rich spa water is available as a liquid iron tonic, as are iron-rich solutions/tablets obtained from plant sources (herbal tonics) which are more gentle on the stomach and may act more quickly.

Vitamin C increases the absorption of inorganic (non-haem) iron when taken at the same time, so it is a good idea to wash down supplements with fresh fruit juice.

Magnesium

Magnesium is the fourth most common metal in the body, and is needed for the function of over 300 enzymes, including those involved in immunity and healing. Dietary sources include beans (especially soy), nuts, whole grains (although if these are processed they lose most of their magnesium content), seafood, dark green, leafy vegetables and chocolate. Drinking water in hard-water areas is also an important source.

Lack of magnesium is common and may affect as many as one in ten people. Symptoms associated with magnesium deficiency include loss of appetite, nausea, fatigue, weakness, muscle trembling or cramps, numbness and tingling, loss of co-ordination, palpitations, hyperactivity and low blood sugar. It can also lead to diarrhoea (in early deficiency) and constipation (in later deficiency). Many of these symptoms are also linked with Candida hypersensitivity syndrome.

Taking a magnesium supplement is a good idea to correct any lack – although it may be better to absorb this through the skin by rubbing on a magnesium-rich oil rather than taking oral supplements. Some people have found that oral magnesium seems to trigger their Candida attacks (for example with itching around the back-passage). If this is the case for you, try using a rub-in oil on your arms or legs instead, from which magnesium is absorbed straight into the blood stream, by-passing the intestinal tract.

Dose

The EU RDA for magnesium is 375mg daily. People who are physically active need more than those who are not as large amounts are lost in sweat. The upper safe limit for long-term use from supplements is suggested as 400mg per day.

High doses of magnesium have a laxative effect, which is desirable in some cases - Epsom salts have remained a popular 'cleanser' since Victorian times, for example. The UK Expert Group on Vitamins and Minerals carried out a risk assessment on magnesium in 2003 and concluded that taking 400mg/day supplemental magnesium would not be expected to result in any significant adverse effects. However, the average magnesium intake from food is around 280mg per day. Drinking water can also contain high levels of magnesium in some areas, and the maximum intake from food, plus supplements, plus water has been estimated at 1400mg per day which will have a significant laxative effect. If this occurs, then reduce or stop the dose.

Magnesium citrate is most readily absorbed, while magnesium gluconate is less likely to cause intestinal side effects such as diarrhoea at higher doses. Another option is to take the coconut-derived antifungal supplement, caprylic acid, in the form of magnesium caprylate for double the benefits.

Selenium

Selenium is a trace element that is so important for health that it is incorporated into proteins as selenocysteine, an amino acid. Selenocysteine is found in at least 25 human proteins and is needed for normal cell growth and immunity.

In parts of the world where soil selenium levels are low, the incidence of serious viral infections (and of cancers) increases. These risks are even higher if intakes of vitamin E and vitamin A are also low. The production of antibodies has been found to increase up to thirty fold if supplements of selenium and vitamin E are taken together.

The best food sources of selenium are Brazil nuts, fish, poultry, meats (especially game), wholegrains, mushrooms, onions, garlic, broccoli and cabbage.

Did you know? *Lack of selenium is a growing cause for concern. The mineral content of crops and livestock depends on the soils in which they are grown. During the last ice age, selenium was leached out of the soil in many parts of Europe, including the UK. While we used to obtain good amounts from wheat imported from America and Canada, our wheat is now mainly sourced from Europe, and our selenium intake fell dramatically between 1978 and 1994 from 60mcg/day to 34mcg/day . As a result, UK blood selenium concentrations also fell by around 50% between 1974 and 1991 as intakes were only half the reference nutrient intake .*

Research

Selenium stimulates the production of a type of natural killer (NK) cells which fight infection. Immune cells from people with low selenium levels are significantly less able to kill Candida yeasts than those whose selenium status is optimal.

Lack of selenium is also recognised as a 'driving force' for viral mutations which may explain why so many new, pathogenic influenza viruses emerge from Asia, where selenium intakes are among the lowest in the world. Influenza viruses recovered from selenium-deficient people consistently show genetic changes in the genes coding for viral proteins. Whether or not the same is the case for yeast infections is currently under investigation.

> *Did you know?* *Selenium-containing shampoos are highly effective at treating skin yeasts that cause dandruff.*

Deficiency

Problems that may be due to selenium deficiency include age spots, pale finger nail beds, increased susceptibility to infection, premature wrinkling of skin, poor growth, subfertility, arthritis, high blood pressure, coronary heart disease, cataracts, pancreatitis, muscle weakness, hypothyroidism and some cancers. Selenium is important for healthy muscle fibres, including those found in the heart. In parts of China, selenium intakes are low enough to cause a form of heart failure (Keshan Disease) and an unpleasant, deforming type of arthritis known as Kashin-Beck disease. These risks seem to be even higher if intakes of the antioxidant vitamins A, C and E are also low.

Dose

Usual dose is 100mcg to 200mcg daily. Although the upper safe level for long-term use from supplements is suggested as 350mcg, selenium experts do not advise taking this higher dose unless deficiency is proven. Intakes just a little higher can cause toxicity leading to a garlic odour on the breath (from dimethyl selenide), fragile or black fingernails, a metallic taste in the mouth, dizziness, nausea and hair loss.

Although supplements are a good way to boost a selenium shortfall, the best quality ones – in which selenium is body-ready and already incorporated into the amino acid, selenocysteine, are derived from selenium-enriched yeasts. If you are following an anti-Candida diet and avoiding yeast-containing products, opt instead for supplements containing inorganic sources such as selenium selenite.

Zinc

Zinc acts as a co-factor for over 200 metabolic enzymes, and is needed to switch on genes involved in immune and healing responses. In fact, zinc has been described as the most important trace element for immune function as it works within the nucleus of immune cells, switching on the genes needed for a ramped-up response against infection. Mild zinc deficiency is common in women with recurrent vaginal candidiasis as it reduces the ability of scavenger macrophages to absorb and destroy invading yeast cells.

Dietary sources include red meat, seafood (especially oysters), offal, wholegrains (although processing removes most of their mineral zinc), pulses, eggs and cheese.

Zinc is vital for the special senses and zinc deficiency is a common cause of loss of the sense of taste (ageusia) and loss of the sense of smell (anosmia), both of which affect some people with Candida. Luckily, deficiency is easily tested for by obtaining a solution of zinc sulphate (15 mg/5 ml eg Lambert's Zincatest) from a chemist. Dilute according to instructions and swirl a teaspoonful around your mouth for ten seconds. If the solution seems tasteless, zinc deficiency is likely; if the solution tastes furry, of minerals or slightly sweet, zinc levels are borderline, and if it tastes strongly unpleasant, zinc levels are normal.

Research findings

A topical zinc sulphate ointment has been used to boost immune reactions against Candida antigens applied to the skin in the diagnosis of delayed hypersensitivity response to Candida yeasts. Candida extracts were administered to each forearm in 47 adults, with a zinc sulphate ointment immediately applied to one arm, and a zinc-free ointment to the other. In the 24 subjects who reacted positively to Candida antigen, the response was significantly greater in the arm to which the topical zinc sulphate was applied – but only in those patients with a normal zinc level. In those with low zinc levels, the anti-Candida immune response was suppressed, suggesting that lack of zinc may reduce the ability of the immune system to react appropriately to yeasts present in the body.

Zinc supplements have been used medically and found effective at suppressing Candida growth in patients receiving anti-viral drugs (zidovudine therapy) to treat AIDS. Those receiving zinc sulphate supplements showed an increase or stabilization in body weight and an increase of the number of CD4+ immune cells (which are depleted by HIV infection). The frequency of opportunistic infections with micro-organisms such as Candida decreased significantly with 11 episodes of infection over two years in those taking zinc supplements compared with 25 in those not taking zinc.

> **Did you know?** Zinc-based barrier creams (eg Sudocrem) help to soothe skin irritation such as nappy rash and eczema. They are worth trying externally to sooth an outbreak of Candid vulvitis – but test a small amount on the area first to ensure it doesn't sting.

Dose

Recommended intakes for zinc vary from 10mg to 15mg per day. The upper safe level for long-term use from supplements is suggested as 25mg per day. occasionally higher doses are recommended under medical advice – but need to be taken together with copper at a ratio of 10:1 eg 15mg zinc:1.5mg copper). High doses of zinc can cause nausea, especially if taken on an empty stomach.

Artichoke

The leaves of Globe artichoke (*Cynara scolymus*) contain unique substances such as cynarin, luteolin, cynardoside, scolymoside and chlorogenic acid that are highly antioxidant, boost bile production, lower cholesterol levels and promote the growth of friendly, probiotic bacteria in the bowel.

Research

A randomized, placebo-controlled trial involving 20 men with acute or chronic digestive symptoms found that 32 mg artichoke extracts increased bile secretion by over 127% within 30 minutes and by 151% after 60 minutes. Even after 90 minutes bile output was increased by 94% compared with the baseline level. This is beneficial for those whose Candida symptoms include bloating, flatulence, nausea or abdominal pain related to poor fat digestion. These symptoms are often diagnosed as irritable bowel syndrome (IBS). When over 550 people with dyspepsia and 279 with IBS took 640mg artichoke leaf extracts three times a day, with meals, their symptoms of abdominal pain, bloating, flatulence, abdominal pain and constipation significantly improved over a six week period.

Dose

Globe artichoke extracts: 320 mg to 1,800 mg daily, with food.

Side effects of hunger and transient increase in flatulence have been reported. Rarely, allergic reactions may occur.

Do not use globe artichoke if there is obstruction of bile ducts or jaundice, or if you have gallstones, except under medical advice.

Caprylic acid

Caprylic acid is a medium chain fatty acid found naturally in coconut oil, palm oil and breast milk. It has a natural anti-fungal action that helps to eradicate *Candida albicans* from the gut without affecting the level of healthy probiotic bacteria. It is fat soluble, and appears to work by entering yeast cell walls so they disrupt. This makes it effective against both commensal (harmless) yeasts and the invasive hyphae form.

Research findings

Japanese researches assessed the anti-Candida activity of four coconut-derived fatty acids: caproic, caprylic, capric and lauric acid and found they all inhibited Candida yeasts and the formation of invasive hyphae (germ tubes). Caprylic acid was the most effective at very low concentrations.

In patients with urinary catheters who experienced Candida urinary infections, taking either one dose of the antifungal drug, fluconazole, or one dose of caprylic acid both rapidly reduced symptoms, but caprylic acid was described as superior and less expensive.

Dose

350mg to 500mg, once or twice daily, usually with food. Select calcium and magnesium caprylate, which survive the digestive process to reach the colon and, as a bonus, provide additional magnesium.

Co-enzyme Q10

Co-enzyme Q10 (CoQ10) – also known as ubiquinone and ubiquinol – is a vitamin-like substance present in all body cells, where it is used in generating energy-rich molecules. It is especially important for muscle cells – including those in the heart - where the need for energy production is greatest.

After the age of 20, your CoQ10 levels decrease, partly because you absorb it less efficiently from the intestines, and partly because its production in body cells starts to fall. Low levels of CoQ10 mean that cells do not receive all the energy they need. As a result, they function at a sub-optimal level and are more likely to become diseased and show signs of premature ageing. This particularly affects immune cells and is one reason why immunity is reduced by increasing age.

> **Did you know?** Dietary sources of co-enzyme Q10 include meat, fish, whole grains, nuts and green vegetables. It is widespread in the diet, and its name 'ubiquinol' means 'found everywhere'.

Research

CoQ10 acts together with vitamin E to form a powerful antioxidant defence against oxidation. Taking CoQ10 supplements increases the number of antibodies made after vaccination, and also increase the number of certain immune cells to boost immunity.

Candida albicans needs co-enzyme Q10 to make energy, just like your cells. Researchers have found the presence of Candida yeasts in the gut leads to competition for available CoQ10, so that you need to take higher doses than usual to obtain a therapeutic blood level (the yeasts can get all they need from your food!)

In 2001, researchers suggested in the journal, Medical Hypotheses, that data from a pilot study using two pathogenic strains of *C. albicans* supported the theory that gut candidiasis hinders the availability and therapeutic effects of CoQ10. This could be of clinical significance for some people – especially those with muscle weakness and fatigue, and those advised to take co-enzyme Q10 supplements to help reduce statin side effects, or to improve a high blood pressure or the muscle weakness associated with heart failure. For those with Candida and fatigue, supplements are definitely worth trying.

Dose

The optimal dietary intake of CoQ10 is unknown. Average adult dietary intakes of CoQ10 are estimated at 3mg to 5mg daily for meat eaters and 1mg daily for vegetarians.

I usually suggest a dose of 100mg (ubiquinol form) or 200mg (ubiquinone form). If you are on a statin drug, higher doses may be needed if you are experiencing muscle-related side effects.

CoQ10 is best taken with food to improve absorption as it is fat soluble.

Cranberry

Cranberries are sour, red berries that grow on small shrubs (*Vaccinium macrocarpon*) native to North America. Traditionally, cranberries were used as a poultice to dress wounds, and to prevent or treat scurvy due to their high content of vitamin C. As long ago as 1968, it was found that Cranberry juice has a significant antifungal effect on skin fungi, which was thought to come from its marked acidity (pH 2.8). More recently it was recognized that cranberry extracts contain substances known as anti-adhesins, which prevent Candida yeasts and some pathogenic bacteria (E.coli) sticking to cells, so they are less able to gain a foothold in the body. Cranberry extracts are also thought to bind iron locally so that it is unavailable for Candida metabolism.

Research findings

When conditions are right, Candida yeasts form biofilms that cling to the lining of the mouth, urinary and genital tract, as well as coating dentures and urinary catheters. Yeasts isolated from people with Candida infections form strong biofilms in artificial urine, and are associated with increased drug resistance.

Cranberry extracts significantly reduce biofilm formation in all *Candida albicans* strains tested, and this action is additive to that of antifungal medication.

In a pilot study, the anti-Candida activity of urine from 31 healthy adults was tested before and after taking cranberry supplements (100mg concentrated extracts three times daily). The acidity of all samples was adjusted to the same level and then incubated with Candida yeasts for 48 hours. The study found significant anti-Candida activity in the urine of 17 out of the 31 volunteers, with significant reductions in the number of Candida yeasts growing in their samples.

Dose

Cranberry juice: 300ml (25% strength) daily for treatment; 200ml for prevention. Cranberry extracts: 500mg daily

NB. If you think you may have a urinary tract infection, seek medical advice – especially during pregnancy.

Curcumin

Curcumin is an orange-yellow antioxidant present in high concentrations in turmeric root – a curry spice used in Ayurvedic and Chinese herbal medicine. Curcumin has powerful anti-inflammatory, immune-boosting and antifungal actions.

Research findings

In one study, curcumin completely inhibited the growth of a variety of foodborne fungi, and all Candida yeasts tested under laboratory conditions. Its antifungal actions against Candida included inhibiting hyphae development and triggering early yeast cell death. Recent research suggests that curcumin protects against Candida infection by inserting itself into host cell membranes to stabilise them and improve the cell's resistance to infection. Curcumin also has a corticosteroid-like action to damp down inflammation and suppress soreness, redness and swelling.

Curcumin also prevents Candida yeasts sticking to lining cells in the mouth, gut and vagina. In fact, a 2009 study that tested the antifungal activity of curcumin against 23 fungi strains found it was significantly more effective than the antifungal drug, fluconazole, in inhibiting the adhesion of Candida species to mouth lining cells.

A cream (Basant) containing a number of herbs including curcumin and Aloe vera was found to have a pronounced inhibitory effect on the growth of Candida yeasts isolated from women with vulvovaginal candidiasis, including three strains resistant to antifungal drugs (fluconazole and amphotericin B). Another study found curcumin extracts were strongly effective against 38 strains of Candida (including those that were resistant to fluconazole).

Curcumin appears to have a synergistic action with the antifungal drug, fluconazole, and supplements are recommended to increase yeast sensitivity to the medical treatment. Laboratory studies show that Candida strains resistant to the antifungal drug become sensitive in the presence of curcumin extracts. It appears to deactivate a membrane 'efflux' pump present in resistant strains that normally stop the drug accumulating inside yeast cells.

Curcumin is used to treat symptoms of irritable-bowel syndrome, which are similar to those experienced by people diagnosed with intestinal Candida. In one study, 207 people with IBS symptoms took turmeric extracts every day for 8 weeks. In those taking 1g per day, IBS symptoms decreased by 53%, and in those taking 2g daily, symptoms improved by 60%.

Curcumin is also used to treat ulcerative colitis, which is sometimes associated with Candida infection. When 89 people with ulcerative colitis (in remission) took either 1g curcumin twice a day or placebo (plus their usual medication) for 6 months, only two out of 43 (4.6%) taking curcumin relapsed, compared with 8 out of 39 (20.5%) taking placebo. Curcumin also improved the findings on endoscopy, suggesting that it is an effective treatment.

Dose

Turmeric supplements can be concentrated and standardised to contain as much as 95% curcumin per dose. Select a product supplying 500–1200 mg turmeric a day, standardized to 95 per cent curcuminoids.

Turmeric may be combined with pineapple extracts (bromelain) to improve its absorption.

173

NB Turmeric increases urinary excretion of oxalates and may increase the risk of kidney stone formation in some people.

Echinacea

Echinacea, or purple coneflower, is a traditional remedy first used by native American Indians such as the Sioux to treat infections and relieve allergic reactions.

Echinacea contains several unique echinacins that stimulate the number and activity of white blood cells responsible for attacking fungal, viral and bacterial infections. It especially stimulates phagocytosis – the process by which white blood cells ingest invading micro-organisms before destroying them. It also contains flavonoids that have an antioxidant action.

Research findings

When white blood cells (granulocytes and monocytes) from healthy volunteers were incubated with two preparations of *Echinacea purpurea* in the laboratory, the migration of white blood cells towards *Candida albicans* yeasts increased by 45% and their uptake (phagocytosis) increased by 30-45%.

Oral Echinacea improves the response to antifungal creams prescribed to prevent recurrent vaginal Candida. In one German study, taking echinacea supplements and applying a medicated cream lowered the recurrence rate of Candida infection to around 16% compared with 60% in women using econazole cream alone.

Dose

160mg to 300 mg one to three times daily. Select products standardized to contain at least 3.5 per cent echinicosides/cichoric acid. Some evidence suggests that extracts processed from fresh (rather than dried) *Echinacea purpurea* plants is most effective.

> ***Did you know?*** *Some sources advise taking echinacea intermittently. This is not necessary. It works by stimulating the activity of white blood cells that absorb Candida yeasts before destroying them. As white blood cells have an average lifespan of just four days in the circulation, this activity is not depleted by taking Echinacea continuously. For those intent on taking it intermittently, immune function remains elevated above normal for several days after taking a dose, so taking it only on week days and not at weekends, for example, should not reduce its effectiveness. If you want to overcome recurrent Candida, however, I suggest taking it continuously.*

Garlic

Garlic (Allium sativum) is such a popular kitchen herb that, worldwide, average consumption is equivalent to one clove per person per day.

Garlic contains a powerful antioxidant, allicin, which is formed when the clove is cut or crushed. This disruption releases an enzyme (alliinase) which interacts with an odourless amino acid (alliin) to form the active allicin.

Black garlic is produced by a natural fermentation process, under carefully controlled conditions of high temperature and humidity. This converts unstable 'smelly' sulphur-containing compounds into stable, odourless substances and also produces a dark pigment, melanoidin. Black garlic is highly prized by gourmands due to its soft, savoury-sweet flavour with molasses, balsamic and garlic undertones.

Did you know? When garlic is cooked, heat inactivates many of the beneficial effects so raw or fermented (black garlic) supplements are preferable to increasing your dietary intake.

Allicin has numerous beneficial effects, including reducing cholesterol production in the liver, relaxing blood vessels and increasing the elasticity of arteries to lower blood pressure, reducing abnormal clot formation and generally improving heart and circulatory health.

For those with recurrent Candida, garlic has beneficial antiseptic and antifungal actions. In the laboratory, garlic extracts increase the activity of immune cells, including macrophages and natural killer cells. This helps to boost immune defences by targeting abnormal body cells and those infected with yeasts, bacteria or fungi.

Did you know? Garlic was known as Russian penicillin after the Russian government used it to treat soldiers during World War II when they ran out of antibiotics.

Research findings

Researchers have found that garlic extracts work at a genetic level by switching off yeast gene activity. This inhibits protein and nucleic acid synthesis in Candida cells and completely arrests the formation of lipids (fats). As a result, the formation of hyphae growth tubes is blocked. Interestingly, allicin reduced the activity of specific Candida genes by a factor of 5.54 fold, which was greater than the antifungal drug fluconazole (3.48 fold). These findings suggest that allicin was at least as effective in suppressing hyphae development in C. albicans as fluconazole, and worked in a similar way, although fluconazole could also suppress yeast growth through another gene pathway.

When garlic extracts were tested against 18 strains of *Candida albicans* and 12 other Candida species, garlic was as effective as the antifungal drug, ketoconazole, in killing all yeasts present.

A paper published in the British Journal of Obstetrics & Gynaecology in 2014 showed that taking garlic extracts reduced the number of Candida yeasts in the vagina of women with recurrent thrush, especially during the second half of the menstrual cycle. Sixty-three women who were culture-positive for Candida species at screening were randomised to take either garlic tablets twice a day, or inactive placebo, for two weeks. During the two weeks before menstruation, daily swabs were taken and the number of live Candida yeasts counted to see how many had more than 100 colony-forming units per millilitre. The number of 'cases' was reduced in those taking garlic (76% versus 90%) with the relative

177

risk reducing by 15%, however this was not statistically significant – possibly because the dose used was too low and the study period too short.

Dose

Aim for at least 900 mg standardized garlic powder tablets a day (either in one dose, or as 300mg three times a day). Look for supplements containing concentrated extracts equivalent to at least 1,200mg (1.2g) fresh garlic (supplying 2mg allicin).

For black garlic, a typical dose is 200mg concentrated extract, equivalent to 2g whole garlic.

Enteric coating of garlic powder tablets reduces garlic odour on breath and protects the active ingredients from degradation in the stomach.

Grapefruit seed

The seed of the common grapefruit (*Citrus paradisi*) were first investigated for their antimicrobial activity when it was noted that they rotted slowly when discarded.

Research findings

Grapefruit seed extracts have a broad-spectrum antibacterial, anti-fungal, anti-viral and anti-parasitic action that is effective against

Candida yeasts and a variety of pathogenic bacteria. They have been used to help clear urinary tract infections and have been used to treat Candida. One laboratory study found that grapefruit seed extracts were as effective as the antifungal drug, miconazole, in inhibiting Candida yeast growth.

NB Grapefruit seed extracts are very different from grapefruit juice, which like other juices is frequently contaminated with yeasts.

Dose

100mg to 300mg daily.

Olive leaf

The olive tree (*Olea europaea*) is well known for the oil of its fruit, but its leaves have a greater medicinal value. Olive leaf extracts have a powerful anti-fungal, antibacterial, anti-viral and antiparasitic activity. Olive leaf extracts are used to treat Candida and other infections and to help overcome fatigue and depression in people experiencing recurrent Candida infections.

Research findings

Clinical studies involving 500 patients suggest that olive leaf is effective in treating 98 per cent of bacterial and viral infections – better than many prescribed antibiotics. The active ingredients are antioxidants (eg oleuropein, hydroxytyrosol) which eradicated microbial infections by interfering with protein synthesis so they cannot grow or reproduce. Extracts also weaken microbial cell walls so they are more likely to absorb water, swell and burst.

A recent study investigating the effectiveness of the antioxidant, hydroxytyrosol, showed it had powerful antifungal activity in the laboratory against medically important yeasts and damaging the cell wall of *Candida albicans*. Even at low doses, it prevented Candida switching to form germ-tubes. *Candida albicans* was killed within 24 hours of incubating in a 15% solution.

Dose

500 mg, twice to four times a day, between meals. For persistent problems take 1 g, three times a day. As symptoms improve, reduce back to a maintenance dose of 500 mg twice a day as necessary.

Peppermint oil

Peppermint (*Menthe piperitae*) is a rich source of essential oils, including menthol, with powerful antiseptic and painkilling properties. Peppermint improves digestion by increasing gastric emptying, stimulating secretion of digestive juices and bile, and also relaxes excessive spasm of the smooth muscle lining the digestive tract. Peppermint is therefore taken to relieve indigestion, colic, flatulence and symptoms compatible with irritable bowel syndrome (IBS) or Candida hypersensitivity

Research findings

When thirty different plant oils were tested for their inhibitory effect on *Candida albicans*, eucalyptus and peppermint oils were by far the most effective, and comparable to the antifungal drug, fluconazole. Other studies have shown that the antifungal activity of peppermint oil is considerably higher than even commercially used fungicides.

A large analysis of data from 12 trials, involving 2,500 people, compared the effectiveness of fibre supplements, antispasmodic drugs and peppermint oil in treating IBS symptoms. Peppermint oil emerged as the most effective therapy with the NNT (number needed to treat) to prevent one person having persistent symptoms was just 2.5, compared with 5 for antispasmodic drugs and 6 for ispaghula fibre. making it the. On average, 75% of people with IBS-like symptoms who take peppermint oil experience a greater than 50% reduction in symptoms compared with 38% taking inactive placebo.

When a solution of essential oils, including peppermint, was used twice daily in the oral care of hospice patients, the number of *Candida albicans* yeasts present decreased significantly compared with patients whose mouths were cleansed with saline, and the degree of oral comfort improved.

Dose

100mg to 200mg (enteric-coated capsules) three times a day, after each meal or as required.

Peppermint oil supplements may produce a warm, tingling feeling in the back passage due to some of the essential oil not being absorbed. This is not harmful and will usually disappear if you cut back on the dosage you are taking.

Siberian ginseng

Siberian ginseng (*Eleutherococcus senticosus*) has been used as a traditional herbal medicine for over 2000 years. It has similar actions to Korean and American (Panax) ginsengs, although it is not closely related and, in many ways is more versatile. Siberian ginseng's unique eleutherosides help to boost immunity enhance vitality and normalise stress hormone levels. As it helps the body to adapt to change, it is often referred to as an adaptogen and is helpful for overcoming exhaustion and tiredness. For athletes, Siberian ginseng improves endurance, and in older people with health problems it has been shown to improve quality of life.

Research findings

Russian researchers have found that Siberian ginseng reduces susceptibility to viral infection such as colds and 'flu by 40%, and that those taking it have a third less sick days from work compared to those not taking it. When 36 volunteers took either Siberian ginseng or placebo for four weeks, German researchers noted a 'dramatic' increase in total numbers of immune cells, especially T-lymphocytes, in those taking the active supplement compared with those on placebo. And, when immune cells (granulocytes and monocytes) from healthy donors were incubated with *Candida albicans*, the ability of white blood cells to absorb the yeasts (phagocytosis) increased by 30-45%.

Dose

1g taken one to three times a day. Choose a brand standardized to more than 1% eleutherosides. Siberian ginseng is best taken cyclically by those who are generally young, healthy and fit. For example, take it daily for two to three months, then stop for a month. Most people begin to notice a difference after around five days, but it should be continued for at least one month for the full restorative effect. Older people, and those who are unwell, may take it continuously.

A few people find Siberian ginseng too stimulating. If it interferes with sleep, take it only in the morning.

CHAPTER 4

Medical Approaches

Anti-Candida drugs mostly work by weakening fungal cell walls so they leak contents, swell with water and quickly die.

Many superficial Candida infections are treated with a topical skin cream, gel or ointment. Candida vulvovaginitis may be treated with a pessary or concentrated cream inserted into the vagina with an applicator, with or without a topical cream for use on the vulva. Another increasingly popular option is to take a single antifungal capsule (fluconazole) by mouth and to also apply a cream for its more immediate, local soothing effect. For recurrent vulvovaginal candidiasis, oral or intravaginal treatments may be continued weekly for six months. More serious systemic (body-wide) Candida infections are treated with oral or intravenous drugs.

This chapter provides details of the common anti-fungal drugs, giving information on possible side effects and who the drugs may not be suitable for. If you develop any side effects that you think may be linked with your medication - even if not listed as possible side effects - always tell your doctor.

NB Do not take any drugs if you are pregnant or breast-feeding, except under medical advice.

Vulvovaginal candidiasis is common during pregnancy and can be safely treated with a topical cream such as clotrimazole. Pregnant women usually need a longer duration of treatment, usually about 7 days, to clear the infection. Oral antifungal treatments are usually avoided during pregnancy.

Topical preparations

With topical preparations, the risk of side effects is small and usually only involves mild burning or irritation - especially when applied to raw, inflamed areas. Treatment should be discontinued if these are severe. Hypersensitivity reactions with itching, redness, swelling and an allergic-type rash occasionally occur but are relatively rare. Some creams may cause weakening of rubber contraceptive diaphragms or condoms so if you use this form of contraception, always check.

NB Always read the patient information leaflet which is supplied with licensed medicines. Many topical treatments need to be continued for three to seven days after symptoms have healed to prevent a recurrence.

Topical imidazole drugs

This group of topical drugs include clotrimazole, econazole, ketoconazole and miconazole. They are applied two or three times a day, and there is minimal absorption from the skin. They are often combined with a mild corticosteroid such as 1% hydrocortisone, to damp down inflammation and provide more immediate relief, especially in sore skin folds. The combination is also helpful when a doctor is uncertain whether or not a mild, localised skin rash is due to a fungal infection or eczema as these conditions are often difficult to tell apart initially.

Some creams should not be applied to broken skin, which is not very helpful when inflammation or boggy skin is present.

Do not use corticosteroid-containing creams long-term, or on the face, as they can cause skin thinning.

For recurrent Candida, intravaginal application of a topical imidazole may be prescribed for 10–14 days, followed by clotrimazole vaginally 500-mg pessary once every week for 6 months. Another popular regime is to prescribe an initial intravaginal topical imidazole for 10–14 days, followed by oral itraconazole (50mg –100mg) daily for 6 months.

Miconazole oral gel (usually a nice orange flavour) is used to treat oral thrush and is used four times daily after meals – retain near the sore areas before swallowing. Treatment should be continued for at least seven days after symptoms have cleared. It can also be used four times daily to prevent recurrence of oral thrush. For those with thrush associated with dentures (denture stomatitis).it may be applied to the fitting surface of dentures, before insertion, for short-term treatment.

Topical polyene drugs

Nystatin is a polyene antifungal used to prevent and treat candidiasis of the skin and mucous membranes. It is both fungistatic (stopping yeast growth) and fungicidal (killing yeasts). It is mainly included in combination creams containing hydrocortisone (anti-inflammatory), dimeticone (water repellent to protect the skin) plus antiseptics or antibiotics. These blunderbuss treatments are excellent for treating moist, boggy infections (eg of skin folds, belly button infections) where they can tackle all the fungi, bacteria and inflammation present for rapid resolution of symptoms.

Nystatin oral suspension (and in some countries, a soft pastille) is used in the mouth, four times daily after food, to treat oral thrush (for seven days - continue for 48 hours after symptoms have resolved). The longer the suspension is kept in contact with the affected area in the mouth, before swallowing, the greater its effect (NB It does contain sucrose). It is not absorbed into the circulation and is usually well-tolerated (see Oral Drugs, below).

Topical allylamine drugs

Although mainly used to treat athlete's foot, ringworm and fungal groin (jock itch) or nail infections terbinafine cream or gel are sometimes prescribed as an alternative to topical imidazoles against skin candidiasis. It works by blocking the synthesis of yeast cell building blocks (eg ergosterol) needed for growth.

Oral Drugs

Recurrent Candida infections often require treatment with oral drugs, especially if there are predisposing factors such as taking long-term antibiotics, diabetes or possibly oral contraceptive use. Any reservoirs of infection that may lead to recontamination should also be treated; including skin and nail infections, the belly-button (you'd be surprised how often it is inflamed), mouth, intestinal tract and the bladder. Sexual partners may also need to be treated (eg with an antifungal cream on the end of the penis) as they can be a source of re-infection even if there is no obvious inflammation of the foreskin.

NB If you need to take an oral anti-fungal drug and are already taking other medications - including those bought over the counter - always check with a pharmacist or doctor that there are no interactions before starting to take the new drug.

Oral fluconazole

Fluconazole capsules are available over-the-counter to treat uncomplicated Candida. It can be used from the age 16 up until the age of 60 years – over this age, it is only licensed for use under medical supervision, to exclude potential health problems in which it should be used with caution.

It is taken as a single dose to treat vaginal candidiasis or male Candidal balanitis in a 150mg capsule.

To treat recurrent Candida, a doctor may prescribe oral fluconazole at a dose of 150mg every 72 hours for 3 doses, followed by 150mg once a week for 6 months.

Candida of the mouth or oesophagus is treated with a lower, 50mg dose, once a day for 7 to 14 days, occasionally extended to 30 days.

To treat invasive Candida infections, and for prevention in immunocompromised patients, it may be prescribed in significantly higher doses, often given in hospital.

Most people don't develop side effects. Those that have been reported with fluconazole include: headache, nausea, diarrhoea, flatulence, rash, and less commonly indigestion, taste disturbance, insomnia, muscle aches, fatigue and allergic reactions. Liver, blood and heart conduction problems have rarely occurred.

Fluconazole should not be taken during pregnancy or breast-feeding.

Oral fluconazole interacts with a number of other drugs including some antihistamines, antifungals, antivirals, anticoagulants and some drugs used to treat epilepsy, asthma, diabetes and heartburn/indigestion.

Oral itraconazole

Itraconazole is active against a wide range of fungi and yeasts, but needs an acid environment in the stomach for optimal absorption. The usual dose for vulvovaginal candidiasis is 200 mg twice daily for just one day.

Itraconazole has been associated with liver damage and with heart failure. It should be avoided or used with caution in people with liver or heart problems.

Possible side effects include: nausea, vomiting, taste disturbances, abdominal pain, diarrhoea, breathlessness, headache and rash. Less commonly, indigestion, flatulence, constipation, dizziness, muscle aches and period problems have been reported.

Oral itraconazole should not be used during pregnancy or breastfeeding. It is important to take proper contraceptive precautions before, during and for 1 month after taking a course of treatment.

Itraconazole can interact with some drugs including antacids and some antihistamines.

Oral Nystatin

Nystatin is licensed for the prevention and treatment of candidal infections of the mouth, oesophagus and intestinal tract. The suspension is also used to prevent oral Candida infection in babies born to mothers with vaginal candidosis.

In the UK, only an oral suspension of nystatin (100,000 units per ml) is available, but in other countries powder, tablets and capsules are available, too.

As a topical mouth treatment, it is held against lesions four times a day, then swallowed (NB it does contain sucrose). It is not absorbed into the circulation from the gut, and passes through, helping to eradicate Candida on the way. It works by suppressing fungal growth, and by interfering with their ability to stick to the intestinal lining. Little information is available on its effectiveness, however, even in the drug monographs. It appears to have similar effectiveness to oral fluconazole for treating oesophageal candidiasis.

Large oral doses of nystatin have occasionally produced diarrhoea, nausea and vomiting. An allergic rash can occur but this is rare.

Intravenous drugs

Echinocandin anti-Candida drugs (anidulafungin, caspofungin and micafungin) or amphotericin are used in hospital to treat invasive or widespread candidiasis, and are given by intravenous infusion. They are mentioned here as reassurance that stronger life-saving drugs are available to treat Candida when infections get out of hand.

Bibliography

Some of the sources used while researching this Help Yourself Guide include:

www.ncbi.nlm.nih.gov/pubmed A comprehensive searchable list of medical research papers.

Watson CJ et al. Associations with asymptomatic colonization with candida in women reporting past vaginal candidiasis: an observational study. European Journal of Obstetrics & Gynecology and Reproductive Biology 169 (2013) 376–379

Shankar AH & Prasad AS. Zinc and immune function: the biological basis of altered resistance to infection. Am J Clin Nutr 1998;
68(suppl):447S–63S.

Netea MG et al. An integrated model of the recognition of Candida albicans by the innate immune system. Nat Reve Microbial 2008. 68-78

Moyes DL & Naglik JR. The Mycobiome: Influencing IBD Severity. Cell Host & Microbe 2012. 11:550-552

Kumamoto CA. Inflammation and gastrointestinal Candida colonization. Curr Opin Microbiol 2011. 14(4):386-391

Zwolinska-Wcislo M et al. Are probiotics effective in the treatment of fungal colonization of the gastrointestinal tract? 2006. J Physiol Pharmacol 57(Suppl 9)35-49

Dismukes WE et al. A randomised, double-blind trial of nystatin therapy for the candidiasis hypersensitivity syndrome. 1990. NEJM 323(25):1717-23

Santelmann H & McLaren Howard J. Yeast metabolic products, yeast antigens and yeasts as possible triggers for IBS. Eur J Gastroenterol Hepatol 2005; 17(1):21-26

Middleton SJ et al. The role of faecal Candida albicans in the pathogenesis of food-intolerant IBS. Postgrad Med J 1992. 68:453-454

Nieuwenhuizen WF et al. Is Candida albicans a trigger in the onset of coeliac disease? Lancet 2003;361:2152-54.

Catassi C et al. non-celiac gluten sensitivity: The new frontier of gluten related disorders. Nutrients 2013. 5:3839-3853

Schulze J & Sonnenborn U. Yeasts in the gut: from commensals to infectious agents. Dtsch Arztebl Int 2009. 106(51-52):837-42

Lenz P et al. Prevalence, associations and trends of biliary-tract candidiasis: a prospective observational study. (Gastrointest Endosc 2009;70:480-7.

My Other Books

Overcoming Gallstones, Medilance Publishing, 2014

Nutrition: A Beginner's Guide, OneWorld, 2013

Eat Well, Stay Well, Connections, 2013

Live Longer, Look Younger, Connections, 2012

Death: A survival Guide , Quercus, 2011

Cut Your Stress, Quercus, 2010

Essential Guide to Vitamins, Minerals and Herbal Supplements, Right Way, 2002, 2010

Cut Your Cholesterol, Quercus, 2009

Natural Health Guru: Overcoming Arthritis, Duncan Baird, 2009

Natural Health Guru: Overcoming Asthma, Duncan Baird, 2009

Natural Health Guru: Overcoming High BP, Duncan Baird, 2008

Natural Health Guru: Overcoming Diabetes, Duncan Baird, 2008

Diabetes Cookbook for Dummies, Wiley, 2007

Menopause for Dummies, Wiley, 2007

Thyroid for Dummies, Wiley, 2006

Arthritis for Dummies, Wiley, 2006

Natural Approaches to Diabetes, Piatkus, 2005

Intimate Relations; Living and Loving in Later Life, Age Concern, 2004

The IBS Diet, Thorsons, 2004

Daily Telegraph Complete Guide to Menopause, Robinson, 2003

Eat to Beat High Blood Pressure, Thorsons, 2003

Live Better: Relaxation, Duncan Baird, 2003

1001 Facts about the Human Body, Dorling Kindersley, 2002

Energy Boosters Handbook, Dorling Kindersley, 2002

Eat to Beat IBS, Thorsons, 2002

A Child's World (Channel 4 series), Headline, 2001

The Total Detox Plan, Carlton, 2000

Simply Relax, Duncan Baird, 2000

Saw Palmetto – Natural Prostate Relief, Thorsons, 2000

Pregnancy – The Natural Way, Souvenir, 1999

Increase Your Sex Drive, Thorsons, 1999

I Want To Have A Baby? KyleCathie, 1999

The Ultimate Stress Buster, Vermilion, 1998, 2003

Super Baby, Thorsons, 1998

The Osteoporosis Prevention Guide Souvenir, 1998

Man Alive: Eating Fit, Marshall Ed, 1997

Man Alive: Better Sex, Marshall Ed, 1997

Menopause, Thorsons, 1997,

Candida, Thorsons, 1997,

Irritable Bowel Syndrome, Thorsons, 1997

High Blood Pressure, Thorsons, 1997

Body Facts Pocket Guide, Dorling Kindersley, 1996

Endometriosis and Fibroids, Vermilion, 1995, 1998

Beating Heart Disease the Natural Way, Galen, 1995

Factopedia: chapter on Human Body , Dorling Kindersley, 1995

The Complete Book of Men's Health, Thorsons, 1995, 1999

Planning a Baby? Vermilion, 1995, 2004

The Hypochondriacs' Dictionary of Ill Health, Headline, 1994

The Body Awareness Programme, Bantam, 1994

What Worries Women Most, Piccadilly Press, 1993

The Bluffers' Guide to Sex, Ravette, 1987-2014